THE FUTURE OF HEALTH CARE

Accompanying titles

The Health Debate Live
The Health of the Nation
The Future of General Practice
Audit in Action

THE FUTURE OF
HEALTH CARE

Articles published in
the *British Medical Journal*

Published by the British Medical Journal
Tavistock Square, London WC1H 9JR

First published 1992

ISBN 0 7279 0742 5

The following picture sources are acknowledged:

Front cover, Stammers and Thompson, Mark Clarke, and Will and Deni McIntyre, Science Photo Library; pages 10 and 18, Hulton Deutsch Collection; page 26, Monitor Syndication; page 61, National Perinatal Epidemiology Unit, Oxford; page 66, Sally and Richard Greenhill; page 78, Melanie Friend/Format.

Typeset by Bedford Typesetters Limited, Bedford
Printed and bound in Great Britain by
Latimer Trend & Company Ltd, Plymouth

Contents

Page

Introduction   ix
RICHARD SMITH, MFPHM, *editor, British Medical Journal,
BMA House, London WC1H 9JR*

Re-examining the fundamental principles of the NHS   1
J B L HOWELL, FRCP, *professor of medicine, Southampton
General Hospital, Southampton SO9 4XY*

Setting a strategy for health   8
ALWYN SMITH, FFPHM, *chairman, Lancaster Health
Authority, Lancaster LA1 3JR*

Which model for delivering care?   16
K A M GRANT, FFPHM, *chief executive, City and Hackney
Health Authority, London EC1A 7BE*

Accountability and the NHS   24
DAVID J HUNTER, PHD, *director, Nuffield Institute for
Health Services Studies, University of Leeds, Leeds LS2 9PL*

Rationing   32
CHRIS HEGINBOTHAM, MA, *fellow in health services
management, King's Fund College, London W2 4HS*

Management and information   44
CYRIL CHANTLER, FRCP, *clinical dean, United Medical and
Dental Schools of Guy's and St Thomas's Hospitals,
London SE1 9RT*

Research, audit, and education   56
NICK BLACK, FFPHM, *senior lecturer in public health
medicine, Health Services Research Unit, London School of
Hygiene and Tropical Medicine, London WC1E 7HT*

Funding health care in the United Kingdom   63
CHARLES NORMAND, DPHIL, *professor of health policy,
Health Services Research Unit, London School of Hygiene and
Tropical Medicine, London WC1E 7HT*

Agenda for health: an economic view   71
    CAM DONALDSON, MSC, *deputy director, Health Economics*
    Research Unit, University of Aberdeen, Aberdeen AB9 2ZD

Manpower   76
    STEPHEN BREARLEY, FRCS, *consultant surgeon, Whipps Cross*
    Hospital, London E11 1NR

Introduction

Health services everywhere are in turmoil. The main driver of the turmoil is the widening gap between what medicine could do given unlimited resources and what can be afforded. But many other factors are also accelerating the rate of change: more and more people, including politicians, are beginning to understand that health is not the product of health services and is actually influenced only a little by what happens in health services; consumers are insisting on more say in health and community services; strategic thinking has come into fashion; populations are aging rapidly; medical technologists are innovating ever faster and more ingeniously, but almost paradoxically health service researchers are increasingly realising that much of what health professionals do is based on the shakiest of scientific evidence; managers are expanding their influence within most health systems; and the expectations of both health professionals and patients are changing.

In such a world it is hard to stay ahead. Mostly individuals and organisations are forced to react to changes that they have not foreseen. The way out of this predicament is to take the long view—to try to look over the problems in front of your eyes to the problems and opportunities that lie ahead. That is what this book tries to do.

The book has grown in a sense from the frustration that doctors and others have experienced in constantly having to react to changing circumstances. The BMA council decided that it would like to try to develop its own ideas and get ahead of the problems, and a small working party was established to begin the process. The working party, of which I was a member, decided that it could contribute most by trying to identify what would be the key issues in health over the next 20 years and asking questions about those issues. One of the ways that it did this was to conduct interviews with a great many people involved in the health debate, and most of those interviews are published in an accompanying book—*The Health Debate Live*.

Identifying key issues and asking broad questions should be a useful contribution, but the working party recognised that its report, *Leading for Health*, was a beginning not an end. The BMA is responding to the report by inviting its divisions to produce motions to be debated at a special large meeting, and over 500 motions have been produced. The *BMJ* responded by asking recognised experts to produce papers on the main issues thrown up by *Leading for Health*. The contributors were encouraged to think broadly and deeply, and the resulting papers are gathered together in this book.

I am writing this introduction at a time when Britain is about six weeks away from an election, and as a result people are reluctant to think even two months ahead. Depending on which party wins the election, the changes that have occurred in the National Health Service in the past couple of years may be thrown into reverse. In response to such uncertainty people may understandably decide to concentrate on the next patient, the next decision, or the next five minutes. To look further ahead may seem a waste of time.

But actually, I would argue, this is just the time to look still further ahead, because whichever party is in power the problems of health, health services, community care, and the educational and research endeavours that underpin them will remain. Indeed, these are mostly such central and difficult questions that they are applicable in all developed countries. This is a book that looks to the future, and some circumstances will change to make some of the statements look dated. But I would bet an oilwell to a zloty that most of the problems will be as relevant at the end of the century as they are now.

RICHARD SMITH
Editor, British Medical Journal

Re-examining the fundamental principles of the NHS

J B L HOWELL

The BMA's agenda for health states that "progressively the high principles of the caring services have been eroded."[1] While it is true that in recent years the ability of the NHS to keep pace with the ever increasing demands on it has been reduced, I see no evidence of erosion of the underlying principles as stated in the NHS Act 1946: "It shall be the duty of the Minister of Health . . . to promote the establishment . . . of a comprehensive health service designed to secure improvement in the physical and mental health of the people . . . and the prevention, diagnosis and treatment of illness. . . . The services so provided shall be free of charge, except where any provision of the Act expressly provides for the making and recovery of charges." The act never promised that the NHS would be either all inclusive or totally free of charge.

A key word in the present context is "comprehensive," which is sometimes assumed to mean all inclusive; but the definition of comprehensive is "comprising much; of large content or scope." Clearly the NHS remains comprehensive within this definition; it never has provided nor ever could provide for every conceivable need.[2]

Providing an adequate health service

Has the range and quality of care in the NHS fallen below the public's expectation? Is care being denied to anyone who has a

1

reasonable chance of benefit? Certainly this has sometimes occurred: some people wait excessively long times for treatment; a child in Birmingham could not get cardiac surgery until the secretary of state intervened; haemodialysis was rationed in the 1960s; organ transplantation is still limited. But in comparison with the totality of care provided by the NHS these deficiencies are few and far between. It is not the range of care that is limited, rather it is the length of time some people have to wait that is the problem. We cannot be satisfied with the present service, yet equally, concern that at any moment a decision may be made explicitly to reduce the range of care provided by the NHS is unjustified.

Concern about providing an adequate health service is not limited to the United Kingdom. Similar concerns are being felt worldwide, ranging from those countries that have so little national and individual income that they can support only the most rudimentary of health services to affluent countries such as the United States, which despite spending more than 12% of its considerable gross domestic product on health does not provide care for millions of its citizens. Public concern in the United States was recently expressed in a cover story of *Time* magazine which recommended changes to the systems of health care.[3]

The question posed by the BMA therefore is timely: Can we maintain equal access to an NHS which provides a comprehensive, good quality service to all in need, largely free at the point of delivery? The question has been focused by the NHS Act 1990, which has made the work of the NHS more explicit than at any time previously.

Can we afford a national health service?

The ability of the NHS to meet its goals is certainly thought to be under threat because in recent years we have not been matching rising demand with corresponding additional resources and the gap between the two until recently has been widening. While we cannot control advances in medical knowledge and technology, we can influence the allocation of resources. A key question therefore is why more money is not being made available. Have we reached the limits of our ability to pay more for our health service? I think not. Between 1948 and 1980 expenditure on the NHS in England (and presumably in Wales and Scotland also) increased on average by about 4% per annum after correction for the effects of inflation (fig 1). This seems to have been sufficient to meet rising demands and to avoid major crises. Extra-

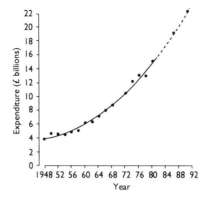

Figure 1—After 1986 rate of increase was increased substantially but gap of about £0·5bn per annum remained in 1990

polation of the best fit curve beyond 1980-1 shows the level of funding expected if the same rate of increase had continued. But in reality, starting in 1980-1 there was a striking reduction in the rate of increase in funding to about 1% per annum and the gap between expectation and allocation rapidly widened. This lower rate continued for several years, during which time health authorities were required to make cash savings and cost improvements while still coping with ever increasing demands for health care. Clearly this could not continue indefinitely and after a few years, as problems became more widespread, the rate of funding was increased (fig 2).

Because the economic fortunes of the United Kingdom over this period did not change abruptly the reduction in the rate of increase in funding between 1981 and 1985 must have been a positive decision rather than one forced on us. What might have been the reasons?

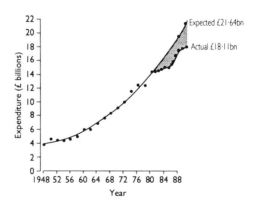

Figure 2—Expenditure on NHS in England between 1948 and 1980 corrected to 1986 prices by annual retail price index.[2] Best fit curve is extrapolated to show expenditure expected if annual rate of increase (4% compound) had been maintained. Between 1980 and 1986 rate of increase slowed to about 1%, with stippled area showing gap between expected and actual expenditure

3

Firstly, the reduction was consistent with the government's policy of limiting the growth of public expenditure. Secondly, there is the "bottomless pit" concept—that is, we will never be able to meet all of the needs of the health service no matter how much money we put into it; therefore we shouldn't try. Thirdly, doctors are sometimes perceived as being arrogant, self interested, and unaccountable and not the best advocates for increased resources. Fourthly, and most importantly, was the perception, until recently, that the resources already provided were not being used efficiently or effectively, that waste abounded, and that extra demands could be met by improvements in the way existing resources were used.

Efficiency and effectiveness in the NHS

There have been many changes designed to improve the efficiency of the NHS. There were two major reorganisations of structure in 1974 and again in 1982, but there is no evidence that they made any significant difference. Perhaps the biggest change in this respect occurred in 1983, when Sir Roy Griffiths was asked to review the management structures in the NHS.[4] He pointed out that consensus management, which had been introduced in the 1974 reorganisation, meant that no one individual was in charge of anything. His recommendation that general management should be substituted was immediately accepted and implemented.

There was one important omission from this constructive report: while Sir Roy described in some detail how general management should be applied to the provision of the resources to the users, it stopped short of recommending how it should be applied to the management of the use of the resources by the users, the clinicians. Sir Roy identified the importance of doctors being involved in management, but without any existing models to draw on wisely did not attempt to recommend how this complex and sensitive process should be done. He did, however, focus attention on this deficiency and in the following year clinical directorate systems were introduced, first at Southampton General and Guy's Hospitals, and subsequently at many other hospitals.[5] This development has been crucially important to the management of clinical resources of hospitals and to instil confidence that resources are being managed and efficiently used.

But despite all of these structural and managerial changes crises of funding continued to occur and led eventually to the prime ministerial review and the major reforms which are embodied in the NHS Act

1990. The essence of the reforms is the separation of the functions of purchasing health care (by health authorities) from the provision of care by providers (the acute hospitals, community units, etc), the two being linked by "contracts." This has shifted some of the power to prescribe how resources will be allocated from doctors (and nurses) in favour of managers and health authorities, and this is widely accepted. It is also recognised that only doctors and nurses acting as general managers can really manage the use of the resources. It is abundantly clear that the efficient running of the NHS requires a willing partnership between professional activity and management.

"Consensus rationing"

The NHS reforms are geared to better management, more accountability, and better value for money; there is nothing in them that implies explicit rationing of care, yet this is now a widely held fear. Why? Simply because many people seem to think that we cannot continue to provide additional resources to meet all reasonable health care needs. Support for this view has been lent by the recent controversial decision of the North East Thames Regional Health Authority explicitly to exclude five categories of treatment from their responsibilities. Further afield, the state of Oregon in affluent America has already introduced legislation to ration care explicitly by denying some categories of patients treatment under the largely state funded Medicaid programme.[67] Further, some of our own health economists are promoting quality adjusted life years (QALYs) as a basis for allocating resources to the more cost effective procedures, and, by implication, high cost and low QALY procedures should not be funded if resources are limited.

One advantage of this form of "consensus rationing" is that it removes from the individual doctor the possibility of conflict with his or her fundamental ethical responsibility of making decisions only in the interests of the patient once he or she has accepted responsibility for the patient's care; this is implicit in the Hippocratic oath. He or she does not have to worry whether the cost:benefit ratio is good enough—the community has already taken this decision and the doctor-patient relationship has not been directly compromised.

But can a community come to these decisions with a clear conscience? Can it be confident that its decisions are just? The experience of Oregon is not encouraging. A process of cost-benefit assessment plus community consultation about the "value" of differ-

5

ent treatments resulted in at least one major anomaly: cosmetic breast surgery was ranked higher than treating an open fracture of the femur.[7] The result was so extremely unreasonable that it was unacceptable, but less obvious anomalies would probably pass unchallenged. Assessments made on the basis of costs and benefits, which are poorly quantified, with the ratio then modulated by "value" judgments made by members of the public, do not inspire confidence. By contrast, at present health authorities make decisions about the allocation of resources to different categories of care; doctors decide about allocations to individual patients, taking into account their detailed personal and medical circumstances together with the pressures on local resources. As long as the gap between demand and resources is not wide, there is no inherent problem with this system. Doctors are given the final decision whether or not to treat within the resources available after balancing their two responsibilities, one to the patient and the other to the community. If treatment is not urgent patients may be placed on a waiting list. As long as this option is available the decision is then not whether to treat but when to treat. The size and nature of the waiting list becomes an important "error signal," reflecting the inadequacy of the service provided, and has the potential for influencing the political decision of the size of the allocation to health care. If resources do not match need the choice seems to lie between the "cost-benefit" list and the waiting list. I find the waiting list morally and practically the more acceptable; its power to gain more resources for the NHS has been well demonstrated.

But have we arrived at the stage where we should accept as inevitable the de facto rationing of the waiting list or the more explicit model of the Oregon experiment?[8] If we have not reached the limit of our ability to fund the increasing demands of the NHS the question we should be asking is not how are we going to ration care—that is, how are we going to rationalise denying some patients care, and in so doing destroy the fundamental principles of the NHS. Rather the question should be how can we ensure that an adequate proportion of the gross domestic product is devoted to the NHS to allow it to meet its responsibilities? Also, how can we ensure that what is already allocated to the NHS is used efficiently and effectively? This is exactly what the reforms are about. Now is surely not the time even to think about denying care to anyone. Anyone can solve the problems in this way; the challenge is how to maintain our commitment to the principles of a comprehensive health service when resources are not plentiful and demands are constantly rising.

The way ahead

Before the reforms the structure of the NHS did not ensure accountability and give confidence to those responsible for allocating the nation's resources that the service was being or ever could be run efficiently and effectively. The new structure has the potential for doing so and it is in everyone's interests that it succeeds. This requires that doctors and everyone else in the service do their best to make it work.

An important new requirement of the NHS Act 1990 is that the needs of each community shall be assessed and published annually in the Director of Public Health's report. Health authorities, as purchasers, are contracting provider units—for example, acute hospitals, community units—to provide specified quantities and quality of care, and this is monitored. It will soon become apparent what needs are not being met, and the public will be able to judge whether or not it is satisfied with the level[1] and deployment of funding of their NHS. Once it is clear that more care cannot come from greater efficiency and effectiveness, the only argument against providing more money is that none is available. Who can assert this today when the United Kingdom spends less on health than most countries in the Organisation for Economic Cooperation and Development, our expenditure per capita being on a par with that of the poorer "olive" countries of Europe.

There is no need even to entertain the possibility of denying explicitly defined groups of NHS patients reasonable care in 1992 or the years immediately ahead. The time to consider the approach introduced by the North East Thames Regional Health Authority and by Oregon is when we truly cannot afford to pay for the quality and range of care that we want—but that time is not yet here. We have not reached that point in the NHS after over 40 years of remarkable medical advances —personally, I doubt that we ever shall.

1 BMA. *Leading for health: a BMA agenda for health*. London: BMA, 1991.
2 Thwaites B. *The NHS: the end of the rainbow*. Southampton: Institute of Health Policy Studies, 1987.
3 Condition critical. *Time* 1991 Nov 25:34-42.
4 NHS Management Inquiry. *Report*. London: DHSS, 1983. (Griffiths report.)
5 BMA. *CCSC guidance on clinical directorates*. London: BMA, 1990.
6 Dixon J, Welch HG. Priority setting: lessons from Oregon. *Lancet* 1991;337:891-4.
7 Klein R. On the Oregon trail: rationing health care. *BMJ* 1991;302:1-2.
8 Smith R. Rationing: the search for sunlight. *BMJ* 1991;303:1561-2.

Setting a strategy for health

ALWYN SMITH

The international debate on the need for national health strategies and what they should contain has been proceeding for several decades without significantly attracting the involvement of the medical profession in the United Kingdom. Indeed, the worldwide crisis of confidence in traditional attitudes to the form and content of professional health practice has often seemed irrelevant to British doctors because of our complacent satisfaction with the NHS and our consequent belief that we have little need to be concerned. This attitude has changed with the government's health reforms.

The health crisis

When the NHS was introduced parliamentary and public debate identified a set of objectives more far reaching than the simple one of providing medical care free at the time of use. These were to promote the nation's health; to ensure the equitable distribution of health care; to render the health service accountable to the nation; and to invest the activities and development of the NHS with a sense of purpose. It is disappointing after more than 40 years to examine its record of achievement against these objectives. The nation's health has progressed less well than that of many other countries; there remain serious inequalities in health and access to health care; accountability of the service to the electorate has almost disappeared; and we have only just begun to develop a strategy for the national health. However, the conversion of the government to the notion of a national health strategy is to be welcomed enormously, and the responses of the main opposition parties and of the BMA encourage the hope that the long overdue debate on the politics of health is about to begin. The pursuit of the national health is as important a matter for political debate as the national economy or the defence of the realm.

It is not only in the United Kingdom that there is a preoccupation with health strategies; indeed, we have come to the subject quite late and after many other countries have been pursuing formally stated strategies for a decade or more. The international public debate arose from a midcentury crisis in the progress of public health services that had several identifiable origins:

- Reduced mortality and a reduced birth rate have led to populations with a larger proportion of elderly people, which has in turn halted the crude decline in mortality and increased the prevalence of chronic and often intractable disease

- Demand for health care has grown and most countries have found it politically difficult to match this growth with a commensurate increase in supply

- The traditional view that improved health over the past 200 years was largely the consequence of a more widely available and more scientifically based medical practice is now generally considered to be untenable

- There remain serious inequalities in the global and national distribution of health and of health care

- There has been a general concern about the growing political power of the medical profession and its appetite for resources

- Anxiety over the possibility of new environmental hazards has accompanied the proliferation of industrial innovation and the huge growth in the transport of goods and people.

What is health?

The debate over the development of health strategies includes consideration of the political nature of health and of its determinants. For some, health is a public resource that is necessary as a basis for many other national enterprises. Publicly provided personal health services in this country originated after the shocking discovery that a large proportion of young men were not fit to fight in the South African war. Health may also be seen as a commodity for distribution, requiring some consideration as to how and to what purpose it should be distributed. The World Health Organisation has declared health to be

9

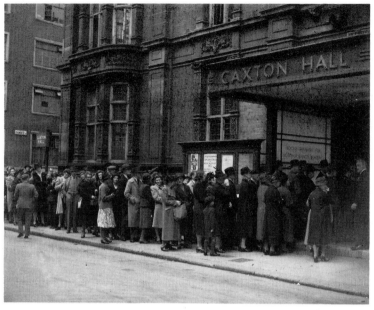

Wartime rationing applied equally to everyone. Can rationing of health care be as fair?

a basic human right—a proposition to which the United Kingdom has subscribed, although many have questioned whether anything can be a right if it cannot be guaranteed. The organisation in an earlier pronouncement has defined health as more than the absence of disease. The difficulties arising from this distinction can be avoided if we quite reasonably define disease as the absence of health, from which it follows that health is the absence of disease.

Some issues emerge quite clearly from the confusions of this debate. It is evident that health is relative—that is, some people are healthier than others. It is also contingent on circumstance—an impairment that would disable a professional athlete might be no more than an inconvenience to most people, and the functional impairments that inevitably accompany aging are quite compatible with a notion of a healthy old age. A useful definition of health is that people are healthy to the extent that they are able to meet their obligations and to enjoy the rewards associated with membership of their community. This definition implies the possibility of two distinct but complementary strategies for the pursuit of the public health. The first entails measures which protect and promote the capabilities of individual people to function in the widest diversity of social contexts. The second entails the development of a society which permits the successful functioning of individual people of the widest diversity of capabilities. Traditionally, we have concentrated largely on a strategy of the first kind—and with some success. What is now required is the concurrent development of strategies of both kinds.

Determinants of health

A strategy for the national health must take some account of the determinants of health, which may be broadly considered under the headings of heredity, environment, lifestyle, services and policies.

Heredity

Heredity needs little consideration, mainly because through evolution we have adapted to a wide variety of environments and most people who survive the neonatal period are well fitted to survive to an old age. Treatment of the minority who incur genetic disease has been one of the more successful developments of clinical medicine. Possibly the most important contribution of heredity to the problems of the public health arises from its role in determining the usual life span of our species and, therefore, the part it almost certainly plays in the genesis of the disease processes by which that life span is eventually terminated in the absence of environmental intervention. The importance of heredity in the aetiology of the diseases of old age may be much greater than has generally been supposed. This would have profound implications for the future pattern of health care.

Environment

Environmental determinants of health embrace both the life sustaining elements whose sufficiency needs to be assured and the life threatening elements whose presence needs to be contained. We need enough and appropriate food, clean water, clean air, and shelter, and the provision of even these basic requirements to all citizens of the world—or even of this country—continues to elude us. We need protection from natural and man made environmental hazards. Our industrial ingenuity contrives to render man made hazards a recurrent challenge.

Lifestyle

Lifestyle as a threat to health is a currently fashionable preoccupa-

11

tion as well as politically controversial. Any attempt to formulate national policies in relation to lifestyle seems to provoke considerable reaction (in both the general and the political sense). The individual's right to choose is invoked against the encroachment of the "nanny" state. The government's stated policy has been to ensure that individual choice is informed and not to influence choice.

We cannot, however, assume that the free and informed choice of individuals would always be for the healthy option, and risking one's health—for example, by smoking, binge drinking, and sexual promiscuity—cannot be generally condemned by any state that may call up people to fight in a war or by people who look favourably on those who risk their lives in sporting activities.

Reaction tends to assume that individual choice is free. This seems most improbable. For example, the national diet has changed profoundly even in the present century. This is not simply the aggregate of individual choices but a reflection of the availability and pricing of foodstuffs and the effects of marketing designed to promote what is profitable to the producers and distributors of food. These in turn are the consequence of political policies governing the use of subsidies and other devices in pursuit of economic objectives. It would not be a new intrusion on individual liberty for these policies to be guided in the interests of the national health.

Services and policies

The originators of the NHS were largely driven by a desire to increase access to health and medical care. Almost from its inception, however, the preoccupation of those responsible for managing it, at both the national political and the local administrative levels, has been with the control of that access and even with its restraint. It would have been politically difficult in the early years of the service, in the aftermath of the privations of war, to be explicit about the need to ration care, but the word "rationing" is now openly used, even by politicians, in debate about the NHS. There is a general acceptance that demand for health care inevitably exceeds supply, and undoubtedly such a mismatch has been increasingly evident over the past 20 years or so. Management of the resulting situation has been largely delegated to the periphery, and indeed mainly to clinical judgments about priorities. As these tend to be based on urgency there has been an increasingly evident neglect of the less urgent but more numerically and socially important care needed for chronic, progressive, and disabling disease and for the prevention of illness and the promotion of health.

A more explicit rationing procedure has become a central issue of the debate about the provision of treatment and care. Unfortunately, many of the realities of rationing have yet to be confronted. The wartime rationing of food, fuel, and clothing was successful mainly because it was generally understood to be necessary and had to be universally applied. For wealthy people to purchase these goods beyond the rationed allowance was not only punishable as a crime but generally condemned as immoral. If health care were to be rationed in the NHS—for example, by the adoption of a restricted list of available procedures—it is difficult to see how we could prevent the use of the scarce resources—mainly staff—for procedures unavailable in the NHS but available for payment in what would be likely to be a growing commercial market.

There are other difficulties in the development of a formal rationing system for health care. Perhaps the most intractable is that of identifying a principle and associated criteria by which procedures would be admitted to or rejected from the approved canon. Two conflicting approaches require consideration. Economists tend to see it as axiomatic that we should seek to maximise the surplus of health benefit over service cost. To that end they urge the use of the mean added years of good quality life as a selection criterion. An alternative objective might be the reduction of health variance, a policy which would seek to provide most care to those most ill. The economist's approach sees the health care system as an element of the national productive economy; the alternative sees it as an element of the national apparatus of justice. Either is a defensible approach: only political debate will lead to an informed national choice.

A national health strategy

A national strategy for health would ideally be based on an explicit national health policy in which the importance of health alongside other national goals such as defence, economic growth, education, and transport is appropriately stated. The weight to be given to health implications in the formulation of these other policies will also need to be considered. We must acknowledge not only the importance of other goals but also the choices that need to be made when health aims conflict with other aims—for example, when industrial safety conflicts with economic competitiveness as in the issue of the European Community social chapter. These are important political questions requiring overt debate.

It is also important to be clear about the part which the pursuit of health should play in national policies. For example, should health be seen primarily as an economic output which we should seek to generate as efficiently as possible for a given resource input or is it a commodity for distribution to individual people? If it is for individuals do we seek to distribute it as equitably as possible or do we favour its unequal distribution as part of the system of differential rewards that may help to drive a competitive economy? Do we agree with the World Health Organisation that the highest attainable level of health is a basic human right, and are we prepared to restructure society so as to redress the disadvantage that derives from impairment of capacity—in other words, to discriminate positively in favour of the sick instead of compounding their disadvantage as at present?

Whatever answers to these questions are to drive the national health strategy, they need to be politically debated. Equally, the detailed objectives of the strategy need to be based on the best possible assessment of their feasibility and be subject to continual monitoring and revision in the light of changing policies, needs, and technical opportunities. There will be a need for appropriate structures and procedures for achieving this both locally and nationally.

Conclusion

The NHS as it has remained for over 40 years and through a series of upheavals, has always lacked both the resources and the remit to adopt more than a reactive role in relation to the demands made on it by patients. A case may be made that the national health is too important to be left to the NHS or to the professionals who work in it, but they remain the principal repositories of the technical and scientific knowledge on which a feasible strategy will need to draw.

For those concerned about the adequacy of health professionals and the present health service the challenge is to contribute not only to the formulation of a health strategy but also to its continued appraisal and development at national and local levels. This may require a reversal of existing policies which tend to isolate the NHS from national and local politics and to restrict its role to the marketing of procedures. The objectives of the government's recent changes included the containment of public expenditure on health services and to that end the limitation of the medical profession's power to consume resources. If we seek to influence the national health strategy we shall have to begin by recognising the weakness of our present position and our need to develop a more productive relationship with the political process.

The views expressed in this article are my own and do not necessarily reflect those of Lancaster Health Authority.

Which model for delivering care?

K A M GRANT

If someone was asked to design the perfect health care system they might come up with the following ingredients. It would be free at time of need to the whole population. It would have as its foundation a high class system of primary care with a gatekeeper role into the secondary care sector. The secondary care sector would be pyramidal in shape with its base consisting of district general hospitals serving populations of 300 000-500 000. These hospitals would deal with the conditions that such populations would throw up in sufficient volume on a regular basis; they would be backed up by regional centres covering larger populations and dealing with patients with less common conditions, referred by the district general hospitals, so that fewer centres would be needed to attract the number of cases needed to run a cost effective service. The whole system would be centrally planned, using, in particular, access to capital and medical manpower as controls to make sure the strategy of the centre was adhered to and there were no unplanned developments or expansion.

The United Kingdom in theory had such a system—the result of a combined effort of two unlikely allies, Nye Bevan and Enoch Powell. Bevan in 1948 set out the principles of free access and universal coverage. Powell, as minister for health in the early '60s, introduced rational planning of health services and the concept of district general hospitals and regional centres.

Changes in the system

Why was such a system changed? Indeed, has it changed as far as the public are concerned? Are the arguments that are polarising health

16

care workers more about the way they wish to work rather than the way the system actually works? For undoubtedly the biggest debate at the present time is about how health care should be delivered. The politicians, including medicopoliticians, may well leap on the more obvious changes, such as NHS trusts and general practitioner fundholders, to make a point, but the fundamental debate concerns the separation of the purchasing and providing roles in health care and the different models of running both of these functions.

The BMA's agenda for health does not attempt to answer these questions.[1] Rather, in its section on models of delivering care, after capturing the main variations in four models—one of planned provision and three concerning the purchaser-provider split—it raises the following key questions: "Is it advantageous to separate the purchaser and provider function? Or could the old planned health care system be improved to a point where it worked better than such a system? What are the relative merits of the two systems? If a purchaser-provider system is preferred which [of the three] model[s] would work best? How can community care best be fitted into such a system?"

Any attempt to answer these questions must look at what went wrong with the old system and whether it is capable of responding to treatment. In particular, is the only treatment necessary more money?

The running of the NHS

No comprehensive scientific study has been carried out into the overall running of the NHS, at least not one that examined both financing and delivery. Many studies have looked at particular aspects of the NHS. Several key points emerge from these:

● The system did not start from scratch. As a result the distribution of hospitals (and their funding) did not always align with the current population distribution

● Regional referral centres were based on hospitals linked with medical schools. Again they did not necessarily fit easily into the NHS structure. London, for example, though serving only four regions, had 12 medical schools, which produced 30% of the country's medical graduates

● The medical manpower system was not perfect. Putting aside the problems of running a pyramidal training structure, this structure did not (and probably could not) tackle the question whether doctors who had a large part of their training in regional referral centres could

17

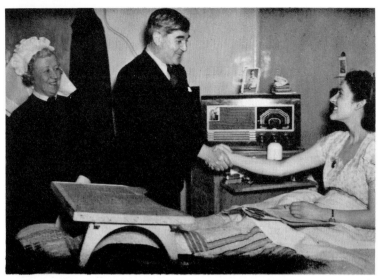

Nye Bevan's principles of free access and universal coverage for the health service still stand as ideals

practise what they had learnt when appointed to district general hospitals. This form of training is perfectly understandable but it might not be either the best use of resources or best in terms of outcome. Training for cancer treatment and for neonatal care are the obvious examples

● Control on capital was not absolute. Fundraising and, more recently, joint ventures with the private sector meant that the introduction of new technology slipped out of the hands of the Department of Health and the regional health authorities

● Capital as a whole was insufficient, in particular to cope with the movement of populations and the development of mental illness and handicap services

● The system was increasingly complex and of necessity bureaucratic. Standard terms and conditions of service for staff, be they in Inverness or London, did not fit well with the complexities of the employment market in the United Kingdom in the '80s. Monitoring the efficiency of the various parts of the services from the centre became impossible. The 1600 "performance indicators" lay largely ignored in the computer disks dispatched from the Department of Health.

Clouding issues

Above all revenue was almost certainly insufficient, but proper debate was obscured by three key factors. Firstly, because patients never had to be billed the true costs of individual patient care were not known. This allowed politicians to duck the issue by pointing out "they must be inefficient, they don't know what things cost" and to compare different hospital costs without taking into account case mix, again assuming that there were still large amounts of cash to be released.

Secondly, the politicians were assisted in their arguments by being able to point to population based data on health status such as perinatal mortality rates and standardised mortality ratios to suggest that in terms of outcome the health service stood up relatively well to international comparisons. They were allowed to confuse improving the health of the population with providing a service whose prime function, as seen by that population, was to treat them when they were ill.

Thirdly, and probably the key to the whole dilemma faced by the NHS, is that the rationing of health care that has been increasingly carried out over the past three years had been carried out previously, if not in secret then in private. Certainly waiting lists were public knowledge, but what was not known was that many people did not even get on to waiting lists. This became particularly relevant as new but expensive technologies came on the scene, starting with renal replacement therapy, when those who were not judged to be "best bets" for a treatment programme were not told "sorry we can't afford it," but "here are some tablets," and they would quietly go home and die. The problem gathered pace in the '70s and '80s with such treatments as angioplasty and joint replacement.

Looking to the future

In summary, what has to be addressed in either revitalising the old system or setting up the new system is how to:

• Recognise the differences and the interrelationships of improving the health of a population as opposed to providing a service to treat people when they are ill

• Provide equal access to the primary and secondary care services while balancing the costs of relocating hospitals and staff with expecting patients to travel

- Relate costs to activity and outcome so that politicians, health care professionals, and, above all, the public can make valid comparisons of efficiency and effectiveness
- Allow changes in service provisions, especially new developments and the introduction of new treatments, to be controlled by those funding the health service—namely, the public or its representatives
- Ensure that when decisions are taken to ration health care that they are taken in such a way that they are open and that the public is aware of them
- Manage such a system with minimal bureaucracy.

Planned provision v purchaser-provider split

Both a system based on planned provision and one based on a purchaser-provider split could deliver these objectives. The question is which is most likely to? In the end it will probably boil down to a view of human behaviour and belief in what is achievable in a system which as long as it represents a very significant proportion of central government expenditure will always be controlled and indeed manipulated by politicians for their own ends.

The problem is it is not possible to experiment. You have to have one system or another. You cannot have some hospitals funded centrally and in effect free goods while others depend on the market, or some parts of the country funded on the basis of their population and the rest on the basis of history, albeit with a planned move towards funding based on the population.

You could look elsewhere. Again this will be unhelpful. All health care systems, be they market based, centrally planned, or a combination, have both successes and failures that proponents and opponents can point to. They are all without exception failing to meet either the public's expectations or governments' wishes to contain cost.

I favour separating the purchasing and providing roles. They are both big roles. Identifying health care needs and allocating resources to meet them require different skills from those required for running hospitals and community services. In particular, if it is accepted that choices will have to be made because demand will always exceed supply then the task will become doubly difficult. Whatever organisation makes these choices will need to take the public with it, so they should therefore be made at as local a level as possible. The centre can also have an input. Together they can plan just as effectively as before if not more effectively. By removing responsibility for providing services the purchasers not only can concentrate solely on purchasing decisions but also will not be bound by loyalty or history and can make decisions objectively. The London regions, for example, might well not have required Professor Tomlinson to advise on their future if those responsible for looking after the residents were not also those responsible for the hospitals.

Similarly, if providers have to concentrate only on providing a service there will be no inbuilt incentive to withhold from the patient what treatment is suitable. There will be no possibility of collusion with managers to slow the system down or ration care without telling the patient. Obviously the money may not be there to meet the need, but the providers' role in advising the patient will be much clearer. There is obviously the risk that excessive, unnecessary, or unproved treatment will be given, but that would assume that the purchasers were weak and this may any way be less harmful than the under-treatment that goes on at present.

Again the question of whether planned provision or a purchaser-provider split is the best model for health care cannot be answered scientifically, but exposing the rationing that goes on can only be for the good of the public if not for the good of the politician and it will be orchestrated only by a purchaser-provider split.

Planning *v* market forces

The next question is whether movement across the purchaser-provider divide should be governed by market forces or planned. If purchasing authorities are strong then they will use the evidence of costs and quality emerging from the provider units to plan their services. The debate centres on whether they will have those skills of analysis and whether or not energy should go into bringing all hospitals up to standard rather than rewarding those doing well. Again it comes down to personal beliefs, especially in human nature. My view is that all the evidence to date of the use of centrally derived performance indicators to improve performance is that they do not work and that the quickest way to expose and change variations in health costs and outcome is to expose them to the public and their advocates, be they district health authorities or general practitioners, and reward those who do well.

21

Fundholding GPs *v* district health authorities

This leads on to the last question: who controls the purchasing agenda, district health authorities acting as agents for the population as a whole or general practitioner fundholders? The answer has to be both.

Fundholding allows the individual general practitioner to act as a powerful advocate for his or her individual patient. Purchasing authorities — and all models suggest merging district health authorities and family health services authorities — need to look at the population as a whole, and their larger budgets are needed to cope with the risk of rare but expensive procedures. There is no reason why the benefits of both systems cannot be combined by fundholding being organised at district health authority level for all practices with local agreements on what is purchased direct by general practitioners and what is part of block contracts. The main feature is to ensure that as much leverage is put on the provider system as possible, both in long term planning and in management of individual patients. The district health authority if properly run has the leverage for long term planning and the general practitioner fundholder for management. It should be relatively easy to get the best of both worlds.

Community care

Providing and purchasing of community care should be the same as for acute care. Indeed, general practitioners would be in a much stronger position to determine what they wish to provide in the primary care field than a separate community provider. Where the major problem will be, as indeed it always has been, is in the division of responsibilities both for home support and for long stay care between the health service and local authorities. It is a morass at the moment, not only in terms of financial responsibility but also in deciding who should look after whom. Equally dependent or indeed independent patients may be found in NHS long stay wards, local authority part III homes, or private nursing homes. Acute wards have many patients who are waiting for home helps or meals on wheels.

Local authority commissioning

The last model put forward in the BMA's document is that proposed by the Institute for Public Policy Research and would make local authorities the purchasers of health care. Bevan opposed this originally because his experience of local authority health care was bad. Nevertheless, it should be examined not least in terms of whether European views or regions gain force here. A regionalised United Kingdom may well give the opportunity to merge health authority and local authority responsibility for purchasing services. The advantages seem obvious, but so do the disadvantages: health would be a local as well as a political football and the learning curve would be large. Again, whether this is the correct way forward can probably never be determined objectively.

Conclusions

A theoretical intellectually strong case could well be made that the present system is the correct one and that it will work if sufficient money is flung at it. However, there is no hard evidence, to back this up. The only hard evidence is that to date no government has flung sufficient money at it and there is no evidence to suggest that this will change in the future. An American politician once said "All health systems have problems — they always will, there will never be enough money — all you can do is tinker with them so that the public think you are doing something." That is dishonest. The purchaser-provider split almost certainly will be the system which will make it most difficult to deceive the public as to the imbalance between funding and provision, and for that alone it should be supported.

1 BMA. *Leading for health: a BMA agenda for health*. London: BMA, 1991.

Accountability and the NHS

DAVID J HUNTER

At various times throughout its history the NHS has been accused of being both centralised, monolithic, and bureaucratic[1][2] and decentralised, fragmented, and insufficiently accountable.[3] At the centre of this paradox is the dilemma of accountability.[4]

At a formal level the issue of accountability is deceptively clear and unequivocal.[5] Health ministers and their officials in the four health departments of the United Kingdom are accountable to parliament for all that happens in the NHS. The health authorities are the agents of the central department and its ministerial head. But while the theory of accountability may be clear, its practice is decidedly less so.

The chain of command

The vexed issue of accountability has exercised academic observers, former permanent secretaries, and official committees for many years. All are critical of current arrangements. The 1979 Royal Commission on the NHS concluded that "detailed ministerial accountability for the NHS is largely a constitutional fiction."[6] The report described the gap which exists between the formal, detailed accountability enshrined in the constitutional conventions governing the NHS and the realities of managing what in practice amounts to an extremely complex and diverse set of activities.

The present NHS reforms, as with earlier reorganisations, do little to resolve this longstanding dilemma. The white paper *Working for Patients*[7] is at pains to emphasise the importance of decentralised decision making in order to free managers to be more responsive to local preferences and the views of users. The purchaser-provider separation, managed competition, and the notion of money following the patient are intended to achieve these aims.

But the white paper betrays an ambivalence evident in successive NHS reforms when it refers to the "chain of command" operating from the coal face of health service delivery to parliament via the secretary of state for health. It is this chain which threatens attempts to unshackle management from political constraints. Some believe this to be at the root of many of the NHS's difficulties. Sir Roy Griffiths expressed concern about the issue and attempted to solve it in 1983 by creating a management board (now the NHS Management Executive) within the Department of Health so as to engineer a separation between political and managerial accountability "to achieve consistency and drive over the long term."[8] But a neat distinction between political and managerial accountability, sometimes portrayed as a split between policy making and implementation, is not sustainable in practice. Political processes do not generate precise, clear cut objectives or the criteria necessary for effective managerial accountability to be achieved.[9]

Finding a balance

There are other features of the NHS reforms which challenge prevailing notions of accountability. In particular, there is the position of NHS trusts, which may enjoy freedom from local health authority control, though they remain accountable to the secretary of state. If trusts grow in number it will not be realistic for the centre to be directly responsible for them. The NHS Management Executive is currently searching for a solution to this problem that is compatible with current conventions.

A little known report published by the House of Commons Public Accounts Committee in July 1991 nicely illustrates the continuing dilemma in the context of the management of the NHS in Northern Ireland.[10] The committee is unequivocal in its view that as an accounting officer the chief executive of the health and personal social services, Northern Ireland management executive, is personally responsible for the funds voted by parliament and entrusted to his care. The committee was "greatly concerned" by the chief executive's answers to its questions and by his arguments that as "day to day management responsibility had been delegated to the Boards . . . [this] absolved him from being answerable [to the committee] on his full accounting responsibilities, although he accepted that he is responsible for ensuring that the services are provided in an efficient and cost effective way and provide good value for money."[10] The

25

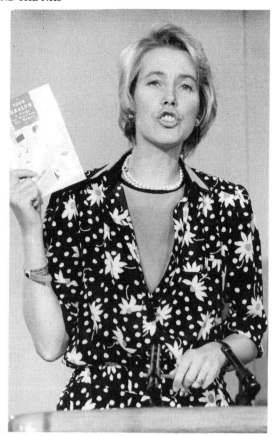

Ministers are
unlikely to be willing
to forsake their
positions of
command in the
health service

committee did not accept the implication that in requiring the accounting officer to discharge his duties it was assuming centralised control of the health and personal social services in Northern Ireland. The committee argued that: "Delegation to others in any large organisation, regardless of management structure or style, or whether the delegated authority is to an agent, in no way removes the requirement for ultimate accounting responsibility to be accepted."[10]

The committee regarded the situation with such gravity that it recommended that the chief executive "should inform the committee within three months of the actions which he considers necessary in order to demonstrate that he is discharging his accounting officer responsibilities."[10] This example encapsulates the essence of the dilemma of accountability, which is to find the optimal balance between top down political oversight on the one hand and devolved managerial freedom on the other. Similar concerns underlie much of the work of the House of Commons Health Committee.[11] It has also been analysed by a former permanent secretary of the Department of Health and Social Security.[9 12]

Little seems to have changed since the infamous phrase in the 1972 DHSS grey book, which set out the management arrangements for the 1974 NHS reorganisation: "Delegation downwards must be matched by accountability upwards."[13] The phrase perplexed observers then and still does. As another former permanent secretary at the then DHSS put it, "No clear prescription was given as to how this [principle] was to be achieved."[14] For Sir Kenneth Stowe the key to the future development of accountability and the NHS lies with parliament, which may need to rethink its role "so as to accept less uniformity, rigidity, and constraint in the bodies for whom it votes resources."[14] It is probably an illusion to expect parliament, and therefore central government, to back off in such a manner while the NHS is funded largely from Exchequer funds.

Given the acknowledged failings of, or, to be charitable, ambiguities evident in, the present arrangements, does a better model exist? Or should we accept the royal commission's verdict that the present system is not without its virtues?

Alternative models

The four alternative approaches appraised by the Royal Commission on the NHS, in ascending order of major disruption to the status quo, were: strengthening the arrangements for monitoring the quality of services, which are the responsibility of health authorities; devolving power to health authorities; establishing a health commission or corporation; and transferring the NHS to local government.

Monitoring quality of service

There have been numerous initiatives aimed at improving and monitoring quality of service, and activity has intensified in recent years. Quality assurance, audit, accreditation, total quality management, medical audit, performance review, and related concepts are all part of the common currency of health service management. There is increasing emphasis on making services more consumer driven rather than profession led, thereby placing a greater emphasis on forms of

27

accountability exercised downwards to local communities. It is a role which has generally been adopted by community health councils, although under the reforms they are no longer the sole channel by which health authorities and managers are expected to communicate with the public. There is now much more diversity as consumer views are sought directly through public surveys, user panels, public meetings and forums, and so on. Whether they offer an appropriate form of accountability exercised downwards to the public is arguable.[15]

Devolved responsibility to health authorities

The royal commission's favoured option was that the direct and detailed accountability for the NHS required by parliament could best be exercised by health authorities themselves. The commission proposed that in England the regional health authorities should become accountable to parliament for matters within their competence.

This proposal has not been enacted for several reasons. Firstly, ministers are reluctant formally to relinquish their power. Secondly, there is continuing uncertainty about the role and functions of regions. Thirdly, the introduction of the NHS Management Executive at the centre has led it to assume central responsibility on behalf of ministers for the operation and management of the NHS. However, it is possible for health authority chairmen and chief officers to be called as witnesses by the parliamentary committees with health interests.

Local health authorities could lead to improved local accountability if members had a legitimate power base in local communities, but they do not.[15] While members, even those appointed under the 1991 reforms, may see their role as more than mere agents of central government it is difficult for them to have legitimate local community accountability when they are appointed rather than elected. However, as noted above, there may be other ways of opening up channels to enable a dialogue to take place with local communities.

Health commission

The suggestion that the NHS be established as a public corporation and become less prone to political interference has generally met with a lukewarm response. The royal commission was equivocal on the issue, neither wholly supporting the proposal nor rejecting it outright. Nor did Griffiths support it in his management inquiry. The general perception is that a major structural change of this kind would achieve little in terms of the NHS enjoying an arm's length relationship with its political masters. Given the vast sums spent on the NHS and the highly political and sensitive nature of health care, it is unreasonable to expect ministers to exercise a self denying ordinance.

The purchaser-provider split offers an opportunity to reconsider the notion of an agency model to provide services while the purchasing or commissioning of services rests with health authorities or newly elected all purpose local authorities (see below). Under the government's "next steps" initiative it would be possible to reconstitute the NHS Management Executive as such an agency with NHS provider units becoming its local arms.[16] The initiative began with the Ibbs report in 1988[17] and is intent on improving the management capability of governmental functions and to distance these from the policy dimension. Of course the issue of accountability would remain to be resolved since, as has been emphasised above, the move to devolved management is no guarantee that the requirements of accountability can be adequately met within prevailing conventions.

Local government option

There are both strong advocates for the local government option[18][19] and committed opponents.[13] The Royal Commission on the NHS opposed it on the grounds that there would be great resistance in the NHS to a local government takeover. But the commission did not rule out local government control over the NHS in the longer term.

A proposal for the local government of health has recently been put forward by the Institute for Public Policy Research.[16] The principal advantages of unitary local authorities are that they would approach their health responsibilities from a wider vision of health rather than from the narrow confines of health services; provide a local democratic base for the articulation and implementation of a broad strategy for health; and end the present division between health and social care which is proving so detrimental to the development of coherent, seamfree community care services.

Under the Institute for Public Policy Research proposals unitary local authorities would function as purchasing or commissioning agencies. They would not be responsible for employing health care professionals, who would operate from NHS provider units managed by the management executive, which would function as a "next steps" agency. This would remove at a stroke the longstanding opposition by NHS doctors to becoming local government employees.

Conclusion

Of all the proposed models only the last confronts the issue of accountability in a way that truly challenges current orthodoxy and firmly shifts the focus of attention from the national to the local level. None of the other proposals gives grounds for believing with any confidence that central interference can be avoided. Local government control of the NHS through purchase of service contracting contains the seeds of a more effective system of control and of accountability to local communities. The arrangement is less imperfect than the present muddle, in which members of health authorities, in theory the agents of the centre, see themselves as primarily accountable to their local community. It is not the fact of election itself which is the guarantor of effective accountability but the combination of election and control over policy priorities and the services provided through the contracting process.

Solutions to the accountability problem do not reside in structures or local government alone. They need to go hand in hand with a modification of existing processes and practices. In particular, there is the position of parliament and the means of financing health care. If it is inconceivable to envisage a radical shift in the funding basis of the NHS from general taxation, then it is to parliament that we must look for hope of change. Parliament should be less concerned with accountability from the point of view of a narrow focus on fiscal regularity and on resource inputs and more concerned with reviewing the outputs and outcomes resulting from these inputs. So far, it has not shown itself capable of adopting, or being willing to adopt, such a focus.

Assuming that as a society we believe that a vibrant local government is worth nurturing and defending—and there must be doubts given national politicians' dislike of local government—then the case for bringing the responsibility for health within its embrace would seem to be overwhelming. It is unfortunate that this option is furthest from the political agenda.

1 Department of Health and Social Security. *Patients first*. London: HMSO, 1979.
2 Owen D. *Reflections on the royal commission. The Trevor Lloyd Hughes memorial lecture.* 25 October 1979. (Mimeograph.)
3 Committee of Public Accounts. *Financial control and accountability in the NHS.* London: HMSO, 1981. (17th Report, HC255.)
4 BMA. *Leading for health: a BMA agenda for health.* London: BMA, 1991.
5 Day P, Klein R. *Accountabilities.* London: Tavistock Publications, 1987.
6 Royal Commission on the NHS. *Report.* London: HMSO, 1979. (Cmnd 7615.)

7 Secretaries of State for Health, Wales, Scotland, and Northern Ireland. *Working for patients.* London: HMSO, 1989. (Cm 555.)
8 Department of Health and Social Security. *NHS management inquiry. Report.* London: DHSS, 1983. (Griffiths report.)
9 Nairne P. Managing the DHSS elephant: reflections on a giant department. *Political Quarterly* 1983;**54**:243-56.
10 Committee of Public Accounts. *The control of administrative manpower in the Northern Ireland health and personal social services.* London: HMSO, 1991. (32nd Report, HC441.)
11 Health Committee. *The organisation and management of the Department of Health and the Department of Health and Social Services (Northern Ireland): minutes and evidence.* London: HMSO, 1991. (HC409.)
12 Nairne P. Managing the National Health Service. *BMJ* 1985;**291**:121-3.
13 Department of Health and Social Security. *Management arrangements for the reorganised NHS.* London: HMSO, 1972.
14 Stowe K. *On caring for the national health.* London: Nuffield Provincial Hospitals Trust, 1989:44.
15 Hunter DJ. Managing health care. *Social Policy and Administration* 1984;**18**:41-67.
16 Harrison S, Hunter DJ, Johnston I, Nicholson N, Thunhurst C, Wistow G. *Health before health care.* London: Institute for Public Policy Research, 1991.
17 Efficiency Unit. *Improving management in government: the next steps.* London: HMSO, 1988.
18 Regan DE, Stewart J. An essay in the government of health: the case for local government control. *Social Policy and Administration* 1982;**16**:19-43.
19 Association of Metropolitan Authorities. *Local government and the NHS: time for a change?* London: AMA, 1991.

31

Rationing

CHRIS HEGINBOTHAM

All health services ration health care. This truism hides a variety of forms. The United Kingdom health service rations through non-availability, primary care gatekeeping, and waiting lists. The United States service rations partly by income and partly by insurance companies funding either a core group of services or by placing treatment and lifetime caps on the cost of an individual patient's care.

Social insurance schemes such as that in Germany ration through protocol agreements with doctors and by payment for a basic service to which the individual consumer can add by additional contribution. Central and eastern European countries have until recently rationed according to the degree of "cunning" that the individual consumer was able to bring—the key skill was knowing the way around the system and who to bribe. Although that is now changing, old habits die hard.

These main features of each system appear in every system to some degree. The NHS is not immune to abuse; sometimes access to the best possible care—even any care—is by having the right contacts. What the United Kingdom does not have, at least explicitly, is a constrained group of core services, or some form of treatment or lifetime cap on the amount that can be spent on any individual. And the United Kingdom has avoided the worst excesses of the American system. Latest figures put the number of uninsured people in the United States at between 35 million and 37 million,[1] some of whom, it is true, obtain Medicaid benefit but many of whom do not. Even those who are insured may have significant limits placed on the benefits that they may receive for the premiums that they can afford.

The BMA's agenda for health[2] sets out four questions about rationing: Is rationing inevitable? Should rationing be explicit? How might rationing be achieved? Who will make the decisions on rationing? In this article I examine these four questions.

Is rationing inevitable?

The short answer to this first question is yes. Empirical evidence from all health services suggests that rationing takes place either covertly or explicitly and always has done. Beveridge's and Bevan's hope that comprehensive health care free at the point of delivery funded out of taxation would eventually become self levelling was an unattainable dream.

Improvements in access, pharmaceutical innovations, and high technology medicine have steadily increased the cost of health care at an inflation rate well beyond the retail price index. In all countries in the Organisation for Economic Cooperation and Development the proportion of gross domestic product spent on health has increased steadily, though at a differential rate. The United States now spends 12% of its gross domestic product per capita on health care, and even with cost containment measures that figure is likely to reach at least 15% by the year 2000, possibly sooner.[3] Table I shows the wide differentials between countries, though these figures must be compared with those in table II for general purchasing power parities (PPPs) and health care purchasing parities—these show that the United Kingdom is not as far behind the United States or Germany as the broad gross domestic product figures may suggest.

None the less the most striking feature of the health care policy debate, particularly during the late 1980s, has been the desire to find

TABLE I—Proportion of gross domestic product (%) spent on health in various countries in 1980 and 1987

	1980	1987		1980	1987
United States	9·2	11·2	Finland	6·5	7·4
Sweden	9·5	9·0	Belgium	6·6	7·2
Canada	7·4	8·6	Australia	6·5	7·1
France	7·6	8·6	Italy	6·8	6·9
Netherlands	8·2	8·5	New Zealand	7·2	6·9
Austria	7·9	8·4	Japan	6·4	6·8
Germany	7·9	8·2	Portugal	5·9	6·4
Iceland	6·4	7·8	United Kingdom	5·8	6·1
Switzerland	7·3	7·7	Spain	5·9	6·0
Luxemburg	6·8	7·5	Denmark	6·8	6·0
Norway	6·6	7·5	Greece	4·3	5·3
Mean				7·0	7·5

Source: OECD, 1987.

33

TABLE II — Health expenditure and gross domestic product per person ($) for 18 countries in 1980, converted by exchange rates and purchasing power parities[4]

Country	Expenditure on health based on:			Gross domestic product based on:	
	Exchange rates	Gross domestic product purchasing power parities	Medical care purchasing power parities	Exchange rates	Purchasing power parities
Austria	722	607	1 119	10 243	8 612
Belgium	747	596	906	11 877	9 486
Canada	788	853	890	10 792	11 692
Denmark	880	668	894	12 932	9 816
Finland	684	564	1 157	10 800	8 912
France	1 040	839	1 267	12 188	9 839
West Germany	1 065	818	1 108	13 221	10 152
Greece	175	211	388	4 163	5 010
Ireland	480	510	684	5 507	5 854
Italy	479	541	854	7 011	7 911
Japan	569	537	1 118	9 101	8 598
Luxemburg	836	707	1 070	12 703	10 738
Netherlands	988	777	1 168	11 959	9 406
Norway	964	773	1 440	14 118	11 322
Portugal	150	237	502	2 483	3 925
Spain	334	376	544	5 665	6 381
United Kingdom	548	484	907	9 482	8 372
United States	1 089	1 089	1 089	11 446	11 446

effective cost containment measures. The United States has gone through a series of organisational developments with the introduction of health maintenance organisations, preferred provider organisations, and other forms of "managed care."[5] Prospective, concurrent, and retrospective utilisation review is now required of provider organisations by many insurance companies. Clinical audit has become a necessity. Worries about escalating costs led to the development of diagnostic related groups, which are now used for the funding of Medicaid and Medicare (for indigent poor and elderly people respectively) by the federal government.

None of these methods seems to be working, perhaps because of the pluralism inherent in the American system, the litigious nature of society, and the demand by American people for the latest diagnostic or technological intervention. Even with some cost containment through reimbursement for diagnostic related groups, many states, of which Oregon is only the most famous, are looking for other methods of resource allocation.

All forecasts of health care expenditure show an ever expanding demand and exponentially increasing cost function. But there are some hopeful signs. Improvements in surgical techniques are bringing down costs, reducing perioperative mortality, and improving the quality of life. Pharmaceutical developments may reduce the need for surgery. Possibly the cost of certain treatments will reduce in real terms (figure). All in all, however, the answer to the question of

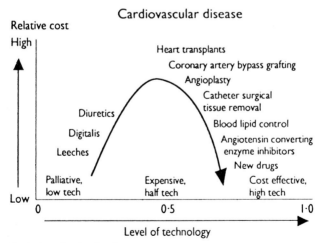

Evolution of technology[6]

whether rationing is inevitable must be a qualified yes. Therefore, the sooner society understands the implications and develops workable approaches the better.

Should rationing be explicit?

If rationing is to occur the next question is whether it should be undertaken by health authorities or provider units without recourse to wider public debate, or whether decisions should be taken only explicitly and openly.

This is not as simple a question as it seems at first sight. There are merits and faults with both covert and explicit rationing. As far as possible any decisions, especially those which have societal and ethical implications, should be public. Not every decision will be taken in the full glare of publicity, especially those about an individual's treatment. Clinicians must be given as wide a freedom as possible to choose the best treatment for an individual patient subject to the patient's informed consent. Yet interventions must be undertaken within a context set by public policy, after public debate about the important organisational, ethical, and social principles on which allocation decisions should be made.

In other words there will be two levels at which rationing is undertaken. Firstly, it will be undertaken at a public level, where broad decisions are made on the amount of money to be put into a particular specialty or subspecialty balanced against the resources available to all other specialties and taking account of health promotion, health prevention, and other methods of achieving health gain in the population. Secondly, it will be undertaken at the level of the allocation of specific resources to individual patients at the point of need by the treating physician. Neither the public, nor health authorities, nor indeed provider managers, can monitor every individual treatment. Insurance companies in the United States are trying to do just that through prospective and concurrent review; but that is in the context of a much more plural and competitive system, which even the reformed NHS is a long way from.

An important development in resource allocation will thus be explicit public policy decision, which narrows clinicians' room for manoeuvre, together with protocols appropriate to certain types of treatment. Both will tighten the boundaries of clinical freedom. Within those boundaries, however, clinicians will retain individual responsibility.

The implications of this are vast. Greater explicitness of the contractual "guidance criteria" may challenge accepted clinical practice or royal college policy and have other unintended consequences also, including an enhanced likelihood of medical negligence litigation.

Rationing is almost certain to become more explicit. The implications of this require a great deal of thought before the more radical health authorities or practitioners open the floodgates to public argument about the resources for every type of illness and the treatment for every individual.

How might rationing be achieved?

Because rationing occurs now and will become more explicit in future attention must be paid to ways in which it can be achieved. A laissez faire attitude will not do. Effective (which includes ethical) priority setting and resource allocation requires: a better understanding of disease and health care needs in the population; a clearer picture of all treatments available and their costs; more detailed information on the effectiveness and outcomes of specific treatments; decisions on the importance to individuals and the population of particular needs being met; and decisions on resource allocation.

These five points raise fundamental ethical, economic, political, social, and organisational concerns. Allocating health care resources is value laden and must incorporate two (sometimes conflicting) concepts: rights to particular forms of care (whether those rights are claimed or are legal entitlements) and utility (the widest benefit for the greatest number in society).

Resource allocation

Resource allocation is often described as the balance of equity and efficiency. Equity refers to equal access for people of equal needs, and efficiency is concerned with achieving the greatest outputs for given inputs. Effectiveness is also important; loosely defined, it is the ratio of outcomes (outputs) to previously established objectives. Health care objectives clearly incorporate the notion of equity. The United Kingdom does not provide specific rights to health care but only a general entitlement moderated by the decisions of health authorities; but similarly there is no formal utilitarian requirement.

A statement in the Health Services Act 1973 says that health authorities must have due regard for the health requirements of the population. Health authorities (with their advisers and in consultation with provider untis) must decide what they believe are the rights to which a local population is entitled, if anything, and what general provision will be made to maximise overall health, or rather to provide as many relevant disease interventions as possible.

Approaches to resource allocation

Several conflicting approaches to resource allocation have been proposed in the past few years. As a generalisation these can be categorised into one of four types:

(1) Purely private systems which create myriad risk pools with different price bands dependent on the health and financial status of the members of each pool.

(2) Systems that rely on marginal change to meet apparent shifts of demand where control on access is through primary care gatekeeping or some other form of initial hurdle.

(3) Managed care or core service groups, whereby conditions treated and treatments available are constrained under insurance or taxation based funding and patients may purchase additional care over and above the basic core group. A special example of these are systems which constrain secondary care to those who have participated in reasonable primary or preventive measures and health promotion activity.

(4) Quality of life or quality of wellbeing schemes, whereby the allocation of resources is made to a list of treatment and condition pairs ranked according to the ratio of cost to the improvement in quality of life produced by the treatment for that condition.

Rationing can be achieved easily. The issue is what is acceptable in a population or culture — ethically, economically, politically, socially, and organisationally. The United Kingdom is unlikely to accept the wholly pluralist approach to health care (as in (1)). Approach (2) is of course exemplified by the NHS. Consequently, if a better system is demanded some variant of approach (3) or (4) is necessary, possibly grafted on to a marginal planning system.

Managed care or core service systems

Many managed care or core service approaches are based on straightforward a priori allocation systems.[7] Usually treatments are divided into relatively homogenous service groups, with known costs and fairly clear quality indicators for an existing service and where there is a known demand (or clearly stated current provision). Only those service groups where an overall increase in benefit might be achieved through reallocation are then considered. Some can be immediately discarded because the treatment is considered indispensable or necessary on either political or economic grounds.

The other service groups are then divided into their main components and the effect of reducing or increasing expenditure is considered. Once a simple decision has been made on changes, quality concerns have to be further considered before the effect of the change in one area is considered in relation to all other areas. This process must be iterated many times but if done carefully and straightforwardly offers a way into making difficult preliminary decisions.

Decisions about which treatments are not for debate and which could be changed are a matter for political judgment or consensus panels, for community conferences and participation, or for expert judgment. What may matter most is that where clear ethical issues are thrown up by potentially radical decisions those concerns are in some way referred to the wider community for further debate.

Several examples of this approach have already appeared in the United Kingdom. North East Thames Regional Health Authority has instructed district health authorities not to purchase a small "basket" of services, including in vitro fertilisation and plastic surgery,[8] which are not clinically indicated.

Sterilisation for men or women is now only patchily available—a victim of health authorities' attempts to reduce the cost of demands that are not life threatening. Because of uncertainties over community care policy some authorities are cutting back on community services, claiming these are not "health" but social care. The danger of this approach is that pure prejudice could influence the choice of conditions and treatment pairs to cut back on.

QALY systems

The second approach to allocation is by using quality adjusted life year (QALY) or quality of wellbeing (QWB) systems. Although quality of life criteria form a core component of systems such as that developed in Oregon[9] (approach (4) above), they can be useful on their own. QALY systems are utilitarian and make judgments about the benefits of treatment in terms of a prospective improvement in quality of life after an intervention compared with the cost of that intervention. The resulting cost per quality adjusted life year can be compared for different treatments for the same condition or various condition and treatment pairs.

39

Categories of care[11]

Rank	Condition and effects of treatment	Examples
1	Acute fatal, prevents death, full recovery	Appendicectomy; treatment for myocarditis
2	Maternity care, including disorders of the newborn	Obstetric care of pregnancy; treatment for low birthweight babies
3	Acute fatal, prevents death, without full recovery	Treatment for bacterial meningitis; reduction of open fracture of joint
4	Preventive care for children	Immunisations; screening for vision or hearing problems
5	Chronic fatal, improves life span and patient's wellbeing	Treatment for diabetes mellitus and asthma; all transplantations
6	Reproductive services	Contraceptive management; vasectomy
5 7	Comfort care	Palliative treatment for conditions in which death is imminent
8	Preventive dental care	Cleaning and fluoride
9	Proved effective preventive care for adults	Mammograms; blood pressure screening
10	Acute non-fatal, treatment causes return to previous health state	Treatment for vaginitis; restorative dental service for dental caries
11	Chronic non-fatal, one time treatment improves quality of life	Hip replacement; treatment for rheumatic fever
12	Acute non-fatal, treatment without return to previous health state	Relocation of dislocated elbow; repair of corneal laceration
13	Chronic non-fatal, repetitive treatment improves quality of life	Treatment for migraine and asthma
14	Acute non-fatal, treatment expedites recovery of self limiting conditions	Treatment for diaper rash and acute conjunctivitis
15	Infertility services	In vitro fertilisation, microsurgery for tubular disease
16	Less effective preventive care for adults	Dipstick urinalysis for haematuria in adults under age 60; sigmoidoscopy for people under age 40
17	Fatal or non-fatal, treatment causes minimal or no improvement in quality of life	Treatment for end stage HIV disease; life support for extremely low birthweight babies (<500 g)

QALYs are valuable in providing numerical information (though this might be spurious) to measure different interventions. Leaving aside criticisms of the initial derivation of the Kind-Rosser matrix,[10] the most serious criticism of QALYs is that they cannot and do not compare like with like when different conditions are concerned. Even within one condition different patients will place varying utilities on similar outcomes. The cost of an additional one year of life, even in substantial pain, may still be a price worth paying for one person (although the cost to the state may be enormous), whereas five years with only moderate pain may not have a high utility for another.

Compound systems

The third approach to allocation was developed in Oregon and has been subject to some unfair and uninformed criticism. This method links a quality of wellbeing scale (QWB), which is not dissimilar to the QALY system, with wider public consultation on what treatment and conditions pairs might be funded. Admittedly, in Oregon this was only for the 20% of health care costs funded through the state Medicaid budget, and so far the scale has had no influence on private insurance funding. Indeed, federal approval to the Oregon scheme has still not been given. After public consultation Oregon listed 17 categories of care in rank order based on a grouping of community values (see box). Condition and treatment pairs ranked on cost and health gain criteria were then fitted into the 17 rank framework. Further consultation was undertaken with the community and professional groups and anomalies were ironed out by an expert panel.[11]

Even with the sophistication of this process mental health, substance misuse, and drug addiction were kept separate owing to the difficulties of handling them in a QALY type system. The QALY and QWB systems are not kind to (or appropriate for) costly long term care for people with continuing and substantial disabilities in comparison with acute interventions for otherwise fatal disorders where treatment prevents death and there is full recovery. Oregon's most recent proposal is to draw the line at number 587 in a list of 709 condition and treatment pairs. As it happens, most of those below 587 are either treatments of very dubious value or conditions that are not life threatening.[12]

The dangers of this system are evident; if funds are reduced the state can draw the line much higher, excluding patients falling within a specific condition and treatment pair. It is strongly utilitarian in that once the decision is made everyone is affected whatever their specific circumstances. But its advantages are equally real. It has forced policy makers to look hard at how they spend scarce dollars; has catalysed a wide public debate; and has provided a model process, if not a final answer.[13]

There is no need for an all out Oregon style approach in the United Kingdom. Most health care is undertaken by the NHS in a culturally very different way to the plural system of the United States. None the less there are those who advocate QALY type rationing systems. Perhaps the best way forward is, as always, a mixture of political, a priori, and empirical decisions using a simple analytical approach similar to that proposed by Donaldson and Mooney.[7]

Who will make the decisions?

The implications of the preceding discussion require resource allocation decisions to be made by a wider group than previously. Clinicians will still have freedom within more clearly defined boundaries or constraints. Those boundaries will in part be set through protocols agreed between clinicians and provider managements with purchasers and will sometimes be enshrined in a contract. The protocols will reflect public policy decisions taken by purchasers after receiving expert and public advice. Expert advice can be obtained from individuals and through expert panels and consensus conferences. Public opinion can be gauged by opinion polls, surveys, public meetings, media debate, and the participation of local and national groups in decision making forums. Doctors will have to accept a wider involvement in decisions on allocation, especially at the macro level. That will put pressure on the micro level of clinical practice, placing greater emphasis on informed consent and possibly defensive medicine.

But at the end of the day the buck will stop with purchaser health authorities, whose job it is to make decisions on behalf of the community subject to sensible negotiation with providers. The medical profession will have only itself to blame if it does not gather effectiveness data and audit information that it is prepared to share publicly. Lack of debate could mean that decisions are made by default which change clinical practice to the detriment of patient care.

1 Ham C, Robinson R, Benzeval M. *Healthcheck, healthcare reforms in an international context.* London: Kings Fund Institute, 1990:61.
2 BMA. *Leading for health: a BMA agenda for health.* London: BMA, 1991.
3 Lamm RD. *The brave new world of healthcare.* Denver: University of Denver, 1990.

4 Parkin D. Company health service efficiency across countries. In: McGuire A, Fenn P, Mayhew K, eds. *Providing health care: the economics of alternative systems of finance and delivery.* Oxford: Oxford University Press, 1991.

5 National Health Lawyers Association. *The insiders guide to managed care.* Washington: NHLA, 1990.

6 Pinto FJ. New paradigms for health care. In: *The economics of health care: challenges for the nineties.* London: Medeq, 1990:17.

7 Donaldson C, Mooney G. Needs assessment, priority setting, and contracts for health care: an economic view. *BMJ* 1991;**303**:1529-30.

8 Ewart I. A family matter. *Health Service Journal* 9 May 1991:18-20.

9 Honigsbaum F. *Who shall live? Who shall die?* London: Kings Fund College, 1991.

10 Rosser R. From health indicators to quality adjusted life years: technical and ethical issues. In Hopkins A, Costain D. *Measuring the outcomes of medical care.* London: Kings Fund, 1990.

11 Oregon Health Service Commission. *The 1991 prioritization of health services.* Oregon: Oregon Health Service Commission 1991:40.

12 Honigsbaum F. In: *Who shall live? Who shall die?* London: Kings Fund College, 1991:48-9.

13 Fox DM, Leichter HM. Rationing care in Oregon: the new accountability. *Health Affairs.* 1991;**10**:7-27.

Management and information

CYRIL CHANTLER

The questions posed by *Leading for Health: a BMA Agenda for Health* on management and information in the health service cannot be answered without considering what sort of service is required to provide health care for the nation. Management arrangements will be influenced by the structure of the NHS and the information required should be determined by the needs of management, medical audit, and health services research.

A national health service

Public funding of health care in the United Kingdom is by no means excessive when compared with that in other countries in the Organisation of Economic Co-operation and Development (table, fig 1) but nor is it extremely frugal. The contribution by individual people from their private income to the total funding of health care remains small in relation to the other countries in the organisation, though it is growing. Publicly funded health services tend to have low costs[1] because the provision of services is controlled centrally rather than market driven and administrative costs are low, particularly if remuneration of professional staff is constrained.

The administrative costs of NHS hospitals with their global budgets were estimated to consume 6·9% of expenditure in 1984,[2] whereas private hospitals billing each patient spend up to 18% of total revenue on administration.[3] Administrative costs are even higher when public money is spent in the private sector because of the need to regulate the use of this money. In the United States administrative costs account for over 24% of expenditure,[4] and most would agree that

Countries in the Organisation for Economic Co-operation and Development ranked in order of public health expenditure per person in 1990 converted to American dollars by using general purchasing power parities

	Gross domestic product	Public expenditure on health
Canada	19 925	1330
Sweden	16 320	1269
Norway	17 799	1226
Iceland	16 194	1201
Luxemburg	18 175	1189
United States	20 774	1089
France	15 568	1022
Finland	15 565	964
Switzerland	18 716	951
Germany	15 943	935
Belgium	14 672	897
Italy	14 727	865
Netherlands	14 609	858
Japan	17 019	830
Denmark	15 452	811
Australia	15 363	801
Austria	14 224	792
United Kingdom	14 907	772
New Zealand	11 822	697
Spain	11 077	573
Ireland	9 858	571
Portugal	7 879	326
Greece	7 643	309
Turkey	4 941	70

the Americans can no longer afford a market driven system,[5] even though their public expenditure on health per capita exceeds that of the United Kingdom (table).

I therefore assume that the United Kingdom, irrespective of which political party is in power, will continue to have a broadly publicly provided as well as publicly financed health care system and that expenditure from the public purse is unlikely to increase sufficiently to finance all the demands that exist. Even countries that spend significantly more than the United Kingdom are experiencing difficulties in meeting the expectations of patients and staff.[6 7] Rationing either in terms of what is provided, to whom it is provided, or when it is provided exists in every health care system in the world. Many countries are currently fundamentally altering their systems by using methods with many similarities to the reforms recently adopted in the NHS.[6 7]

The problem with public services is that they tend towards central

45

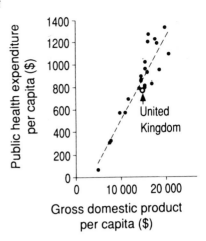

Figure 1—Relation between gross domestic product per capita and public expenditure per capita in 1990 for 24 countries in the Organisation for Economic Co-operation and Development converted to American dollars by using general purchasing power parities

bureaucratic control with an inadequate sensitivity to the consumer's convenience and wishes. Examples of this phenomenon in the NHS abound[8] and were summed up by Polly Toynbee in 1984: "Unless the needs and wishes of patients are catered for soon, I fear that many of them will start voting with their feet, and leave the service that until now they have, in the main, admired and even loved, warts and all."[9]

Clinical efficiency and effectiveness

The management structure of the NHS must be sensitive to patients' needs and encourage clinical efficiency and effectiveness. Clinical efficiency or resource management is vital in a cash limited service and indeed is almost an ethical responsibility because profligacy in the treatment of one patient is likely to lead to denial or delay in the treatment of another. Clinical effectiveness or medical audit is a requirement, firstly, to make sure that the care that we render is effective and, secondly, to ensure that striving to reduce costs does not lead to inadequate standards of care. There are ethical issues involved in this analysis in what is, and always will be, a cash limited service, for where rationing exists the quantity of care available becomes an issue of quality. Perhaps one approach is to define acceptable quality and having achieved it to strive for the maximum efficiency. Information is required for both resource management and medical audit as there are wide variations in costings and mortality for different procedures between different hospitals.[10][11]

A purely market driven system for the delivery of health care is neither possible nor desirable.[12][13] Some planning concerning the delivery of services is essential, particularly in services that require complex high technology with a highly skilled, multidisciplinary team. There is also evidence that better outcomes are obtained with higher volumes for several procedures. Therefore the arguments for some planning encompass both clinical efficiency and effectiveness.[14]

Structure of the NHS

Decentralisation of control

My preferred structure for the NHS designed to satisfy these various considerations would have the following features. Decentralisation of authority and responsibility for the delivery of care with accountability for outcome would be encouraged with doctors and other professionals involved in the management of the service or, in Sir Roy Griffiths's words, "The clinicians mut be involved closely in the management process, consistent with clinical freedom for clinical practice. They must participate fully in decisions about priority in the use of resources."[15] I can see the sense of separating the demand and supply side; according to Enthoven this means that institutions which are independent of the production of services should set standards and priorities, measure achievement, and seek value for money. "Until now," he has said, "the NHS has been a monopoly—as if we said to students 'you can set your own exams and grade them.' "[16]

I would like to see the district health authorities and family health services authorities combine to fulfil this role with some form of local representation and strong links with local authority social services. By agreement, however, some services need to be commissioned from a wider geographical area, perhaps through consortia of district health authorities coordinated at regional level, and capital planning for building and maintenance of hospitals would also be undertaken from the regional level. Decisions concerning the overall allocation of resources made by the district health authorities and family health services authorities would clearly entail setting priorities and determining choices. None the less, the decentralisation of the management of the hospital or provider units to multidisciplinary care groups would allow the groups the freedom to develop their service within a given level of expenditure and still to make choices

47

for the benefit of individual patients. These suggestions are compatible with the recent NHS reforms, which are beginning to show benefit.[16]

Community services

World wide there is a strong movement towards smaller hospitals with shorter lengths of stay and more outpatient investigation and treatment. The development of community facilities for diagnosing and treating minor conditions and for providing care for chronically ill patients is also important. There is certainly a risk that the strict separation of the management of hospitals from community services will delay progress in this area and there are arguments for developing single management structures for community and hospital services. The problem here though is the risk that such organisations will be dominated by the hospitals. The role of the district health authority or family health services authority as the commissioner of services is very important in either model to ensure that community services are developed and resourced and that arrangements exist for integration between the community and hospital services.

Accountability

Accountability for both provider hospitals and for district health authorities would be to the regional authority or office of the NHS Management Executive. Districts would be funded as presently planned according to capitation with adjustments for morbidity, mortality, possibly social deprivation, and the costs of providing services in a particular geographical area.

Cost analysis

In terms of management costs and information required there is a considerable difference between a service which is required to price per item of service and one where costs are analysed to enable valid comparison of hospitals' performance.[17 18] Most of the work of any individual hospital will continue to be derived from one particular district health authority or family health services authority and the relationship between the two would be best described by a service contract specifying the quality and quantity of work to be achieved for a given amount of money rather than the detailed pricing of each item of service rendered. Contracts based on prospective pricing would be reserved for transfers in from other authorities either by contract or as extracontractual referrals. For these cases and for referrals from

Index 1981 = 100

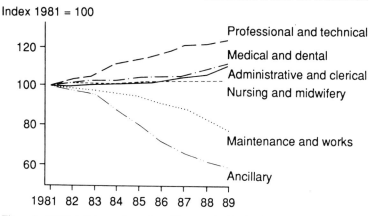

Figure 2—NHS staff in post by main staff groups for England (source: government's expenditure plans, 1991-2 to 1993-4[19])

general practitioner fundholders there would be a national system for grouping inpatient and outpatient care into a limited number (perhaps five to 10) of bands according to the main diagnosis. Significant extra costs caused by, for instance, intensive care or expensive investigations would entail an agreed extra charge. This would not necessarily imply a national pricing system as hospitals could set their own charges for each band. The aim would be to

Index 1978-9 = 100

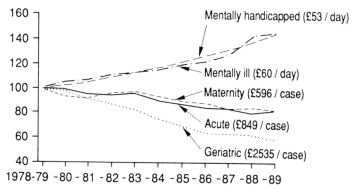

Figure 3—Average costs in 1989 for inpatient day or case and from 1978 to 1986 by type of hospital and by specialty from 1987 to 1989 (source: government's expenditure plans, 1991-2 to 1993-4[19])

49

achieve the benefits of cost analysis in promoting clinical efficiency and effectiveness without the bureaucracy associated with detailed pricing.

Management

Spending

Most people, not only doctors, resent resources spent on administration and argue that more good would result if more doctors, nurses, and other professional staff were employed. Such considerations probably underly the BMA's question: "What proportion of the NHS budget should be spent on management and administration?"

As already discussed, the administrative costs of NHS hospitals are low and figure 2 shows that the increase in the number of professional and technical staff as a proportion of all NHS employees has exceeded that of administrators and clerical staff over the past eight years. The question is really too simplistic, as good management can improve the efficiency and effectiveness of clinical care. Figure 3 shows how the cost of treating patients in hospitals has changed over the past 10 years after allowing for movement in pay and prices in the health service. Reports by the Audit Commission have shown how better management can improve both surgical services and the use of nursing resources.[20][21] At Guy's Hospital between 1985 and 1988 yearly expenditure was reduced by 15% or £8m each year without a reduction in the volume of patients treated.[22] I suspect that the proportion of the NHS budget to be spent on management and administration will vary from hospital to hospital and service to service. If outcomes are compared both in terms of cost and quality of patient care then it will become apparent where changes in the mix of expenditure are required.

Influence

With respect to the BMA's next questions: "What should be the relative influence of professionals, managers and politicians? How may the best balance be achieved? How should they work together? How can professional advice to decision makers be provided?" various models in clinical management have been suggested.[23] The arguments for clinicians participating fully in the management of their services are compelling.[15][22][24] Briefly stated, in a cash limited service everyone has a requirement to maximise efficiency and effectiveness. The quality and quantity of patient care is largely determined by the professionals, particularly doctors and nurses, and it is imperative that they work together to achieve this by pooling their professional expertise rather than patrolling their professional boundaries. Unless they are fully involved in the management process and accountable for its outcome it is difficult to see how this can happen. Proper safeguards to protect their clinical responsibilities to their patients, their time, and their standards are essential.[22] The key is the management team, with the provision of proper administrative support for clinicians with a management role so that they can continue to fulfil their clinical responsibilities. It is important here to re-emphasise that when Sir Roy Griffiths proposed the concept of general management for hospitals he did not intend that "the results should be yet another profession in the National Health Service to work in parallel with other professions"[12]; rather he intended that all who are involved in the delivery of service should contribute to the management of it.

As long as the NHS is almost wholly financed out of taxation it is inevitably and rightly bound to the political process. That process is very much concerned with the allocation of national resources, and it is the function of politicians to reflect and interpret the debate and then to make decisions, which are often very difficult, about how these resources should be deployed. Professionals obviously contribute to the debate and influence the usage of the resources provided for health care within the structure discussed above.

Involvement of health professionals

My answers to the BMA's questions "Should doctors and other professionals be involved in managerial work? How should this be organised and at what level should they work?" will already be apparent. Doctors should be involved at all levels. The nature of their involvement, however, will be different at different levels. At Guy's Hospital the system initiated in 1985[22] continues to evolve. Authority and responsibility with accountability for delivering a clinical service according to a business plan is being devolved down to care groups or teams of doctors, nurses, and others who provide a specific clinical service. Care groups that work within a specialty are coordinated by a management team that provides administrative support. The operational responsibility for the hospital is vested in the management board, which is chaired by a clinician and on which all the clinical directors sit along with the unit manager and functional directors.

51

Clinicians participating in management should be given full responsibility and authority and be accountable along with their colleagues in the management team for the fulfilment of properly constructed business plans. In my view they should resist the imposition of management structures which exclude them or simply involve them in advisory roles.[22]

Information

Expenditure

To outside observers the lack of relevant information for management in the NHS is surprising.[8 10] Considerable resources are now being devoted to changing this. For instance, in 1990-1 revenue expenditure on resource management, medical audit, and information technology totalled £64·7m with another £54·6m devoted to capital in these areas.[19] Certainly the new NHS will require better information systems if it is to be effective.[25] The BMA asked a number of questions concerning information such as: "How much information is needed? What information is required? How may it be most cost effectively collected? How should it be made available and to whom? Where do priorities lie in funding health, administrative, and management information systems?"

Standard systems

It is certainly possible to spend and waste a good deal of money in this area. The cardinal test that we have applied at Guy's Hospital is that the information technology should in the first instance be designed to improve patient care and that, secondarily, the information necessary to analyse costs and quality of care should be gathered through the same systems wherever possible. There is a strong case for a mandatory minimum set of information to be gathered for both inpatients and outpatients, identifying the patient with a unique NHS identity number, date of birth, sex, residence, dates of admission and discharge, identification of the doctor in charge, diagnoses, procedure, and outcome. Such a system should eventually allow the long term outcome of clinical intervention to be monitored and will facilitate the national initiative on health services research. It is also important that management accounting systems are introduced into all hospitals if resource management is to work,[22] and again the systems utilised should be the same throughout the service so that valid comparisons can be made. A lead by the NHS Management Executive in determining national minimum datasets and accounting practices is required.

The NHS is, and should remain, a single service, sensibly decentralised but with clear accountability for performance to the centre. In this respect each part of the service should be required to comply with standard systems where this makes sense. As well as accounting practices and the acquisition of minimum information, standard practices should be introduced to govern transfer of patients between different institutions such as tertiary referrals or extracontractual referrals and, again, the minimum information required for the task should be determined.

New systems

Many of the new information systems being introduced will, or should, improve patient care directly. For instance, the decentralisation of the organisation of outpatient departments with direct booking to the office of the clinician concerned is facilitated by a computerised patient information system for both inpatients and outpatients and aids the preparation of clinics so that all the information required is available at the time of consultation.[22] Such systems can also reduce the amount of clerical work required on the wards from junior doctors and generate standard discharge summaries and outpatient letters. Computer linkage of the laboratories with the wards facilitates the transfer of information, and costing data required for resource management is easily added on to such a system.

Computerised information systems to support medical and clinical audit linked with the total hospital information system are very important. It seems likely that more and more clinicians will be agreeing guidelines for the management of certain types of cases and auditing outcome in terms of deviance from guidelines and success of treatment, both in the short and long term. Such information systems will be necessary if the full potential of health services research in increasing clinical efficiency and effectiveness is to be realised.

To me the acid test is will the expenditure improve patient care and, if not, is it justified? The same criteria can or should be applied to the information that is collected other than that required for the minimum national dataset. Another important criterion is that wherever possible the information should be collected only once and computerised information systems should be judged by the extent to which they allow professional staff to devote more time to patient care rather than clerical work.

The final questions asked by the BMA concerning information relate to the need for health services research to determine the value of clinical interventions. A national system of collecting minimum data for each patient episode as discussed above should provide a very powerful tool to enable the questions to be answered. In the words of John Roberts, "The potential for learning about the effectiveness of various treatments is awesome in a closed medical system such as the NHS, especially with the information technology that the government has pushed and that general practitioners are adopting."[8]

1 Culyer AJ. Cost containment in Europe. In: *Health care systems in transition*. Paris: Organisation of Economic Cooperation and Development, 1990: 29-40.
2 Office of Health Economics. *Compendium of health statistics*. London: OHE, 1984.
3 Parker P. A free market in health care. *Lancet* 1988;i:1210-4.
4 Woolhandler S, Himmelstein DU. The deteriorating administrative efficiency of the US health care system. *N Engl J Med* 1991;**324**:1253-8.
5 Relman AS. The Shattuck lecture. The health care industry: where is it taking us? *N Engl J Med* 1991;**325**:854-9.
6 Ham C, Robinson R, Bezeval M. *Health check: health care reforms in an international context*. London: Kings Fund Institute, 1990: 1-112.
7 Roberts J, Pockley P, Hellema H, Dorozynski A, Bono A, Yamauchi M, *et al*. The politics of health. *BMJ* 1991; **303**: 1011-3.
8 Roberts J. Navigating the seas of change. *BMJ* 1991;**302**:34-7.
9 Toynbee P. The patients and the NHS. *Lancet* 1984;i:1399-401.
10 Smith R. Words from the source: an interview with Alain Enthoven. *BMJ* 1989;**298**:1166-8.
11 Bunker JP. Variations in hospital admissions and the appropriateness of care: American preoccupations? *BMJ* 1990;**301**:531-2.
12 Griffiths R. *Seven years of progress—general management in the NHS*. London: Audit Commission, 1991.
13 Enthoven A. *Reflections on management of the National Health Service*. London: Nuffield Provincials Hospitals Trust, 1985.
14 Black N, Johnstone A. Volume and outcome in hospital care: evidence, explanations and implications. *Health Services Management Research* 1990;**3**:108-14.
15 NHS Management Inquiry. *Report*. London: Department of Health and Social Security, 1983. (Griffiths report.)
16 NHS Management Executive. *NHS reforms: the first six months*. London: Department of Health, 1992.
17 Culyer AJ, Posnett J. Hospital behaviour and competition. *Competition in health care. Reforming the NHS*. In: Culyer AJ, Maynard AK, Posnett JW, eds. London: Macmillan Press, 1990: 12-47.
18 Craig N, Price C, Backhouse A, Bevan G. Medical audit and resource management: lessons from hip fractures. *Financial Accountability and Management* 1990;**6**:285-94.
19 Department of Health and Office of Population Censuses and Surveys. *Her Majesty's government's expenditure plans 1991-92, 1993-94. Departmental report*. London: HMSO, 1991. (Cm 1513.)
20 Audit Commission Review. *A short cut to better services: day surgery in England and Wales*. London: HMSO, 1990.
21 Audit Commission. *The virtue of patients: making better use of ward nursing resources*. London: HMSO, 1991.

22 Chantler C. Management reform in a London hospital. In: Carle N, ed. *Managing for health result*. London: King's Fund, 1990.

23 Disken S, Dixon M, Halpern S, Shocket G. *Models of clinical management*. London: Institute of Health Services Management, 1990.

24 Chantler C. How to be a manager. In: *How to do it*. Vol 3. London: BMJ, 1990:30-9.

25 Smith P. Information systems and the white paper proposals. In: Culyer AJ, Maynard AK, Posnett JW, eds. *Competition in health care. Reforming the NHS*. London: Macmillan Press, 1990:110-37.

Research, audit, and education

NICK BLACK

The limited ability of cost containment strategies to resolve the problems besetting health services is increasingly being recognised. There is a growing awareness among politicians, managers, clinicians, and the public that, while changes in the financial management of health services may help to improve the environment in which care is provided, financial measures do not address the underlying issues of the effectiveness, appropriateness, and humanity of care.

The need for a shift in approach was recognised by, among others, Arnold Relman, when he wrote in 1988 of the dawn of "the era of assessment and accountability"[1]: "We can no longer afford to provide health care without knowing more about its successs and failures. The Era of Assessment and Accountability is dawning at last; it is the third and latest—but probably not the last—phase of our efforts to achieve an equitable health care system, of satisfactory quality, at a price we can afford." If this approach is to succeed a widespread change in attitude on the part of the medical profession will be required. There needs to be a far greater acceptance of current uncertainties in medical practice, combined with wholehearted support for evaluative research. Without this it will prove impossible to place the health service on a firm, scientific base. This does not mean, as defenders of uncertainty are prone to suggest, that the art of medicine is to be sacrificed but rather that wherever possible scientific evidence should be able to be marshalled to suggest that the care being provided is effective. The new era can be achieved only through, firstly, an expanded programme of health services research; secondly, medical audit to ensure research findings are adopted in clinical practice; and, thirdly, education to change some well established professional attitudes towards medicine.

Research

Criticism of previous research

The extent of our knowledge about the effectiveness of medicine is uncertain. David Eddy recently suggested that as few as 15% of interventions have been adequately evaluated.[2] Even if the true figure were twice that, it is clear that our aim of improving the health of the people will prove impossible until more is known about the effectiveness of care. Up until now research has suffered from being almost entirely uncoordinated. With one or two notable exceptions (such as the Medical Research Council's AIDS programme) no attempt has been made to establish research priorities and strategies. As a result the limited resources available have often been wasted on studies which either unnecessarily repeated existing work; were too small to achieve meaningful results; or were methodologically weak, being undertaken (in the true British tradition) by keen amateurs without appropriate scientific training. It has been suggested that only 1% of the articles in medical journals are scientifically sound.[2]

Many of these criticisms may become things of the past. During 1992 we shall see for the first time the emergence of a research and development strategy for the NHS.[3] This offers an opportunity for more relevant and cost effective research to be performed. It should prove easier for the large, multicentre studies that are commonly needed to resolve current uncertainties to be undertaken. However, three factors threaten this optimism: funding for this initiative has still to be secured and there will be many who will resist more being spent on research; the political imperative of regional devolvement may rob us of the opportunity of a national strategy, with the potential to coordinate with similar programmes in other countries; and, as ever, research studies will remain dependent on clinicians' acceptance of their own uncertainty—an attitude that is not always evident.

Specialised and methodological centres

How best can research be organised? We face a long term shortage of high calibre scientists (doctors, nurses, statisticians, economists, sociologists) trained in health services research methods. Both to maximise the productivity from those who are available and to develop expertise in each of the main areas of health care a series of specialised research centres should be established along the lines of the highly successful National Perinatal Epidemiology Unit in Oxford. In addi-

57

tion to these topic focused centres, some methodological ones (such as for clinical trials) to advise on and manage large studies are needed.

Opportunities for researchers

Whatever way the research strategy is organised, it must address several obstacles that currently hamper progress. The first is the lack both of training opportunities and of a career structure for non-medical researchers. The development and funding of masters courses in health care evaluation are needed, along with doctoral training fellowships (in addition to the postdoctoral ones currently provided by the Medical Research Council and the Wellcome Trust). Secondly, there is a need to develop training opportunities for young clinicians who want to enter health services research but in the long term remain in clinical practice: clinical sciences programmes exist in the United States and have produced some first class clinician researchers. Increasingly, opportunities should be provided for clinical registrars and senior registrars to undertake health services research for their doctorates rather than considering only basic science or clinical research, as currently happens. Thirdly, research funding bodies should be more prepared to fund structured reviews of the existing literature; such tasks require experienced, senior scientists and therefore are not cheap, but investment in such work will prove highly cost effective in that it will ensure the funding body identifies an appropriate agenda for future research that should be supported. Finally, even among the more enlightened members of the profession, there is a tendency to believe that evaluative research can be conducted only by doctors who work in the same specialty—for example, only surgeons can carry out research on surgery. While clinicians clearly have an essential and unique contribution to make, we must not lose sight of the fact that they also have a vested interest in the subject of study. Health services research must be independent of bodies and individuals with a particular interest in the topic if a high degree of objectivity is desired.

Dissemination of results

The best efforts to establish a coordinated research strategy will have little or no effect on the health of the people unless the results are disseminated and applied. Dissemination can be aided by the use of structured abstracts for scientific papers and financial support for systematic (rather than opinionated) review articles. The support of professional associations such as the royal colleges is also important.

The real difficulty lies in persuading clinicians to modify their practice in the light of research findings. This is the principal task of medical audit.

Audit

Responsibility

Doctors must take prime responsibility for raising the quality of medical care. That is not the same as ultimate responsibility, which lies with the purchasers of care. Contracting for services is still at a primitive level and largely based on a combination of existing patterns of care and estimated prices. Quality criteria (covering the appropriateness, humanity, and equity of care) will need to be introduced in future years. In theory this will give purchasers the ability to ensure that high quality care is being provided and make doctors more accountable to the public for their actions. In practice this will be achieved only if valid, reliable, and cost effective methods of monitoring quality are developed. This in turn requires more investment in methodological research into outcome measures and process indicators such as readmission rates and hospital mortality. Faced with the danger of losing contracts, provider managers will have to take on the responsibility of ensuring their clinicians are auditing their own work and can demonstrate its high quality.

Defining what constitutes high quality will need to be negotiated by purchasers and providers. This will require one or other party being aware of the relevant scientific literature. Acting on behalf of the public, purchasers will need to incorporate lay people's views of service quality into the negotiations. This will be particularly relevant for aspects of the humanity of care (such as waiting times and the attitude and behaviour of staff). Purchasers are already adopting methods for obtaining the views of the public.

Cost effectiveness

The inclusion of quality criteria in contracts presupposes that clinicians can act to improve quality. Broadly speaking five approaches have been tried: information feedback, education, administrative rules, financial incentives, and penalties. The key finding from evaluations of all five methods is that success is associated with the involvement and support of respected clinical leaders in the specialty. Without them audit may have little or no impact. It is also important

59

to recognise the cost of audit, which may be greater than any tangible benefits that are obtained. This underlines the need for more research that evaluates the cost effectiveness of audit. It is salutary to note that the country which has developed and practised audit the most, the United States, is also the country facing the greatest problems to do with cost containment and overutilisation.

Clearly, the amount of time clinicians could spend on audit is almost limitless. It is therefore necessary for a finite amount to be allocated and priority topics selected, rather than trying to take on everything at once. It is also necessary for routine methods of audit to be developed which do not require vast amounts of medical time. This in turn will require doctors to make much clearer and more comprehensive notes of their clinical decisions and actions so that a non-medical auditor can interpret the care that was provided from the medical records.

Funding

Who will fund audit? If purchasers require providers to demonstrate the quality of care they are providing, then the cost of audit will be included in the contract agreed between the two protagonists. However, purchasers will have great difficulty in interpreting the audit data they are supplied with by providers unless they can compare the information with that obtained from other providers. There is therefore a need for comparative audit databases to be established. Some are already being developed with research and audit funds obtained from national and regional bodies. Should such sources of funds dry up in the future, comparative audit would have to be funded by purchasers. Whether they will is unclear at present.

Education and training

Change in attitudes

Much of what has been suggested above can be successfully implemented only if doctors alter some of their attitudes towards the way they practise medicine. For some this will not be easy. It will entail changing their views of their relationship with patients, accepting greater accountability to their patients and the public at large, supporting the need for more scientific evaluation of medicine, and accepting the need for regular systematic audit of their own work.

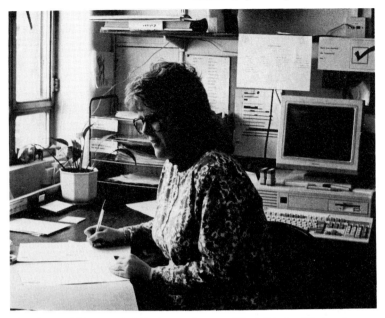

There is a need for more specialised research centres like the National Perinatal Epidemiology Unit in Oxford

Undergraduate education

One place to start promoting the "era of assessment and accountability" is in medical undergraduate education. For years criticisms of the traditional curriculum have been made. In brief, the curriculum tends to reflect the working practices and patterns of teaching hospital consultants, despite the fact that less than 5% of students will end up working in such an environment. Attempts to increase the relevance of the curriculum by introducing more primary care, teaching communication skills, and widening the hospital training experience by incorporating attachments to district general hospitals have all helped. However, many components of courses remain anachronistic, while occupying disproportionate amounts of time. Reductions in these areas would mean that there would be few logistical problems in introducing new areas of learning such as the philosophy of science, scientific methods, medical audit, and management skills. For these are the skills, alongside clinical ones, that the students' future employers are going to value. The primary responsibility of medical

61

schools is to prepare their students for their careers. In the interests of their students, therefore, medical schools must take note of employers' views. Clearly, too great an influence by employers over educational content and standards could potentially be damaging to the health of the public. For example, if the NHS (as the principal future employer) funded medical education some longer term educational objectives might be sacrificed for short term benefits. It is therefore safer to maintain funding of undergraduate teaching by the Department of Education and Science with academic control in the universities' hands.

Postgraduate education

In contrast, funding of postgraduate and continuing education by the NHS is long established, though postgraduate deans derive their authority from universities as well as the health service. Further training has the advantage that the recipients have had experience of the subjects being taught and tend therefore to be highly motivated to learn. This provides an excellent opportunity for medical audit to be teamed up with postgraduate education to their mutual benefit. For instance, the discovery through audit of suboptimal care can act to stimulate interest in a subject and generate a demand for education. In turn, any educational intervention is more likely to be effective if the recipient perceives a need for change.

1 Relman AS. Assessment and accountability. The third revolution in medical care. *N Engl J Med* 1988;**319**:1220-2.
2 Smith R. Where is the wisdom. . .? The poverty of medical evidence. *BMJ* 1991;**303**:798-9.
3 Department of Health. *Research for health. A research and development strategy for the NHS.* London: DoH, 1991.

Funding health care in the United Kingdom

CHARLES NORMAND

The BMA's agenda for health raises a number of questions about the funding of health services.[1] In addition to funding mainly from general taxation, the document considers social insurance, a hypothecated tax, payments and copayments by individuals, private insurance, funding through local government, voluntary contributions, and income generation. It goes on to consider the level of funding for health services and the questions of what is the appropriate level and how that level might best be determined. The third set of funding questions relate to the allocation of the funds over the different health and social care programmes and the factors that should determine the allocation.

Methods of funding

Spending on health care in the United Kingdom was 5·8% of the gross domestic product in 1989[2] and is unlikely to be very different in 1992.[3] Most of this (87%) is public spending on health services.

The countries that are near the bottom of the league table in terms of percentage of gross domestic product spent on health services typically fund services through general taxation (for example, Spain, Denmark, Portugal) and those with higher proportions typically have social insurance arrangements on the Bismarkian model (Germany, the Netherlands, Austria). However, once the level of income in the country is taken into account (and in general richer countries spend higher proportions of income on health), the link between the funding mechanism and the proportion of gross domestic product spent is weak.

In considering the mechanism for funding health services it is useful to start with some principles. These are listed in the box.

63

Principles for funding health services

- The cost of collecting the funds should be low
- The system should be equitable
- The funding should be adequate and not be subject to fluctuations
- The system should not lead to conflict with other government objectives
- The public should be satisfied with the system
- The system should not channel funds into low priority programmes or away from high priorities

Hypothecated taxes

The arguments against hypothecated taxes are that they incur high collection costs; are subject to fluctuations in receipts; and cannot be directly compared with other government programmes, some of which may make a significant contribution to the health of the population. It should be an aim to minimise the cost of collecting the revenue, and if a tax for health were separate from existing mechanisms collection costs would rise. Public enthusiasm for spending on health would probably mean that there would be relatively little opposition to increases in the health tax, which could conflict with the government's objectives in terms of overall taxation and spending.

It is not clear why the government should object if the public chooses higher spending on health services funded fully by higher taxes. In terms of the macroeconomic effects there is no difference between public or private spending on health services of a given amount, and there has been no suggestion that the government should restrict voluntary spending on health. High spending on health will have some macroeconomic effects,[4] but these may be acceptable to the public.

Variations in the receipts arise if a tax has a narrow and unstable base. For example, a payroll tax rises when the rate of employment and wages rise and falls in a recession, when the number of unemployed people rises. Given that health care needs do the opposite, a tax on earnings has problems. A sales tax to fund health services has the same risk of giving falling receipts during recessions.

There are mechanisms that can avoid some of the problems of variations. For example, the tax can be paid from general government funds for unemployed people (as in the new Czech system). It is also possible to vary the rate of the health tax so as to keep the yield constant. However, this conflicts with other government objectives. Increasing a payroll tax or a sales tax during a recession is likely to lead to a fall in demand and a rise in unemployment.

There are also some fears that a special health tax would fall disproportionately on poorer people. There is no reason why this should be so, but taxes such as national insurance in the United Kingdom are regressive (that is, the proportion of income paid is higher for those with lower incomes). It would be possible to devise a health services tax that is progressive if this were desired. In general the issue of equity is best seen in the context of the overall burden of taxation. The present tax system has little progression (that is, the proportion paid by those with high incomes is similar to that for the lower paid).

In summary, in terms of the principles suggested in the box, a hypothecated tax would probably increase collection costs and might lead to fluctuations in yield. It would be more popular with the public, but less popular with the Treasury. The visibility of the payment and the total resources devoted to health services might make patients and providers more aware of the costs of treatment and care. There is no guarantee that the rate would be set at a level that would provide adequate funding—a hypothecated tax is still under the control of the government—but popular pressure could allow selective increases in the health tax.

Social insurance

Social insurance is really a variant of the hypothecated tax. Contributions are on the basis of ability to pay and are not actuarially fair. Its main differences from funding from general or hypothecated taxation comes from different attitudes. Social insurance tends to use the language of insurance, with specified entitlement to specified cover.[5] This contrasts with the more general entitlement to care under most tax funded systems, notwithstanding the patient's charter. It is difficult to be sure whether this difference in attitude is really due to the framework of insurance or to differences in the culture of countries.

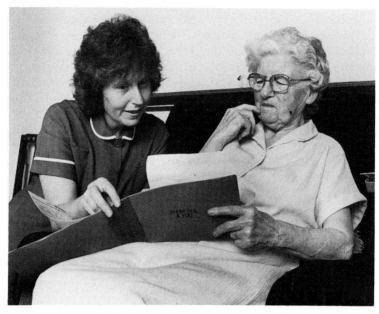

The aging of the population will necessitate increased expenditure on continuing care and treatments for conditions that are not life threatening

Payments and copayments

The argument for direct payment for services by patients is that this prevents use of services where the costs exceed the benefits. Services provided free at the point of use will always have excess demand.[4] However, it is difficult to devise a system of payments that does not also deter people who would benefit significantly. Means testing is inefficient and costly to administer.

It is worth distinguishing two arguments. Firstly, the uncertainty about the need for services by an individual patient means that some form of insurance is needed. This means that government funding or some form of insurance is always likely to be chosen. As with all insurance, copayments can be only a small proportion of the cost in large claims. There is at most a limited role for payments by individual people for high cost services that have uncertain demand by each person. In principle people do not need insurance for health service needs that are entirely predictable, such as routine dental and eyesight checks, as they can predict the costs with certainty and put aside funds for these purposes.

Secondly, the purpose of funding by taxes and social insurance is partly to offer a service irrespective of ability to pay. Payments and copayments conflict directly with this objective. Use of health services has been shown to fall as copayments rise, but demand is inelastic.[7 8]

Copayments can be useful in discouraging frivolous use of services but will never be a source of a large proportion of the funds for health services.

Private insurance and employer based schemes

The arguments against the use of private insurance as the main source of health services funding have been well rehearsed,[14] and the advantages of this system are few. A more interesting question is that of the role of private insurance to supplement public spending. The higher proportion of gross domestic product spent on health in Germany and the Netherlands as compared with the United Kingdom is largely explained by the difference in private funding—that is, spending on services in addition to the government scheme.[26] Germany spent an average of 200 European currency units (ecu) per capita on private health care in 1977, as compared with 89 ecu in the United Kingdom. The Netherlands spent 236 ecu per capita in 1987 on private care.

Funding by employers has a tendency to reduce the level of employment, and leaves those in casual employment and those unemployed without cover. Administrative costs are high, and the source is subject to fluctuations. Employers may offer supplementary medical cover as a tax efficient part of the overall remuneration, but this leads to distortions in the allocation of resources. As a mechanism it has little to recommend it.

There is frequent political criticism that private insurance is interested only in profitable, low cost care and does not cover expensive and unpredictable treatment and care. This is largely true and is likely to continue.[9] In so far as the treatment would otherwise have been administered by the NHS (possibly after a delay), the contribution of the private sector relieves pressure on public funding. There is, however, a risk that the government's commitment to funding will be reduced to take account of the private spending.

In terms of the principles suggested in the box private spending is expensive to collect and administer, conflicts with equity objectives by giving unequal access, and is a fluctuating and unreliable source of

67

funds. If private spending displaces public spending these problems are serious. If it is genuinely supplementary, then the costs fall on those who choose to spend money on private insurance. Tax relief on private policies may increase the contribution by private patients to the cost of their care, but at the cost of devoting government resources to a relatively low priority group.

Multiple sources of funding

The use of several different sources of funding for any overall level of spending means that the costs of administration are high. There therefore should be a prejudice against this approach. The only reasons to choose to use many sources are related to allocation of health services, the possibility of increasing overall funding, and encouraging innovation and diversity. For example, social security funding has allowed the development of different patterns of residential and nursing home care for elderly people. In general multiple sources of funding might be expected to work against efficient resource allocation, but some neglected high priorities may possibly come to light.

Summary of choices

Decisions about the overall level of funding are essentially political. Changes in the mechanism might make health services expenditure more acceptable, and therefore increase the total. It would, however, be unwise to expect resource constraints to be significantly relaxed by changing the funding mechanism. Hypothecated taxes might allow some increase in funding, and, if offered as social insurance, might lead to clearer entitlements to services. A serious danger is that of changing to a funding mechanism which consumes more resources in the process of raising the revenue.

Level of funding

In principle it is possible to define the appropriate level of spending on health services—that is, health spending is a priority so long as an additional pound spent on health services yields greater benefits than it would in other government or private spending. It is, however, difficult to put this into practice.

It would be easier, however, to move towards this type of calculation if better data were available on the costs and effectiveness of health care interventions and other spending options. It is easier to make a case for additional spending on health care if the existing programme concentrates on interventions that are clearly high priorities and additional interventions that offer significant benefits can be identified. The case for higher levels of funding will have to be made on the basis of a demonstration of the cost effectiveness of additional spending.

International comparisons of spending are sometimes misleading as they take no account of differences in the cost of providing services and the efficiency of provision. However, comparisons show that the United Kingdom spends less than the average for other developed industrialised countries, and has held the proportion of gross domestic product spent on health nearly constant over 10 years. There is evidence from opinion polls that the public are in favour of higher spending. Experience in other countries suggests that it is possible to remain prosperous at the same time as devoting a larger share of gross domestic product to health care.

If increases in overall health care expenditure are to be justified on grounds of cost effectiveness many developments will be in continuing care and in the expansion of established treatments for conditions that are not life threatening.[4] The effects of the aging of the population are mainly to increase needs in these areas. It also will not be easy to justify additional funding for those parts of the country that are already relatively well funded until a more equal distribution is achieved.

There is no reason to believe that the present mix of spending on prevention, health promotion, primary care, secondary care, and tertiary care reflects the pattern of cost effective available interventions. Too little data exist to allow these comparisons to be made. Again the principle should be to choose the funding of each level of care to achieve the maximum effect with any level of spending, but it is not currently possible to do this.

I have suggested above that the debate about the level of funding will in future be conducted on the basis of identifying additional, cost effective interventions that have a higher priority than other spending in the public and private sectors. As needs for care grow, with the additional requirements presented by advances in medicine and the aging population, many opportunities will probably exist for identifying high priorities for spending within health and personal social services.[10] Higher spending on health and social care is likely to be acceptable to the public but will bring with it a greater need to demonstrate the effectiveness and cost effectiveness of interventions.

69

1 BMA. *Leading for health: a BMA agenda for health.* London: BMA, 1991.
2 Sheiber G, Poullier J-P, Greenwald L. Health care systems in twenty four countries. *Health Affairs* 1991;**10**:22-38.
3 Robinson R. Health expenditure: recent trends and prospects for the 1990s. *Public money and management* 1991;**11**:19-29.
4 Normand C. Economics, health, and the economics of health. *BMJ* 1991;**303**: 1572-7.
5 Cichon M. Health sector reforms in central and eastern Europe. *International labour review* 1991;**130**:3.
6 Figueras J, Normand C, Roberts J, McKee M, Hunter D, Karokis A, *et al. Health care infrastructure needs of the lagging regions. Report to the Commission of the European Communities.* London: London School of Hygiene and Tropical Medicine, 1991. (Report to the Commission of the European Communities.)
7 Phelps C, Newhouse J. *Co-insurance and the demand for health care.* Santa Monica: Rand Corporation, 1974.
8 McGuire A, Henderson J, Mooney G. *The economics of health care.* London: Routledge and Kegan Paul, 1988.
9 Proper C, Maynard A. Whither the private health care sector. In: Culyer A, Maynard A, Posnet J, eds. *Competition in health care—reforming the NHS.* London: Macmillan, 1990.
10 Bosanquet N, Gray AM. *Will you still love me? New opportunities for health services for elderly people in the 1990s and beyond.* Birmingham: National Association of Hospitals and Trusts, 1989.

Agenda for health: an economic view

CAM DONALDSON

The BMA's agenda for health poses some searching questions on funding of health care: "How much should be spent on the health and community care services? How can that amount be determined?"[1] Unfortunately, the suggested approach to analysing these questions is flawed. In this article I explain why this is the case and what the role of economics should be in setting an agenda for health, in particular in setting the health care budget.

How not to set an agenda: international comparisons

Often, much is made of data on mortality, morbidity, and health care expenditure across countries (usually those in the Organisation for Economic Co-operation and Development (OECD)). An "international comparisons industry" has become established, using such data not because they tell us what we want to know but rather because they're there. The BMA's agenda falls into the same trap. On the one hand the document claims that there is no "'right' amount to spend on the NHS." On the other hand it contains several international comparisons, implying that there is a magic number (of pounds spent on health care) to which all societies should be moving: "If Britain were to bring its expenditure up to the average for OECD countries then about another six billion pounds would be needed for the health service this year."

One problem with such comparisons is that health care is defined differently in different countries. It is well known that one of the reasons why Sweden seems to spend more than the United Kingdom

Health care expenditure per capita, male life expectancy, and perinatal mortality in OECD countries*

	Per capita expenditure (1982) ($)†	Male life expectancy at age 40 (1980) (years) ᐟ	Perinatal mortality (1981)
Australia	798	33·9	1·30
Austria	684	32·5	1·20
Belgium	636	32·0	1·30
Canada	1058	34·0	1·07
Denmark	736	33·9	0·90
Finland	629	31·8	0·79
France	996	33·2	1·23
Germany	883	32·9	1·05
Greece	256	36·4	1·87
Iceland	832	36·5	0·76
Ireland	532	32·0	1·36
Italy	607	33·7	1·70
Japan	673	35·9	1·10
Luxemburg	719	31·3	1·11
Netherlands	851	34·7	1·07
New Zealand	481	33·1	1·05
Norway	822	34·7	0·96
Sweden	1239	34·9	0·77
Switzerland	990	35·1	0·91
United Kingdom	539	32·7	1·20
United States	1388	33·3	1·26

*Source: OECD, 1985.[2] Portugal, Spain, and Turkey are omitted because the data are incomplete.
†Calculated in current dollars by using purchasing power parity exchange rates.

is that Sweden has one of the highest rates of placing elderly people in institutions. Expenditure on these institutions is included in Sweden's total expenditure on health care. So like is not being compared with like.

Even if expenditure was defined similarly across countries, international comparisons would still be flawed. From the 21 OECD countries for which a comparison can be made (table) take Australia, for instance.[2] Some countries spend less than Australia and achieve better health outcomes (for example, Denmark and Japan); other countries spend more but do not necessarily do better on outcomes (for example, the United States and France). Can anything be inferred about the allocation or misallocation of health care resources in Australia? Unfortunately not. The mortality data are crude indicators of health. They are not measures of the potential product of health care. Health care is productive only if it improves mortality or morbidity or prevents deterioration.

The use of international comparisons is naive. Not surprisingly, when based on such methods, a judgment of the effective impact of health care is elusive. It always will be, no matter how good the data are in the future. It is the method that is at fault. We need methods which tell us, within a country, what are the costs and benefits of changing the current uses of health care resources and of expanding or contracting the health care budget relative to other health producing activities.

Setting an agenda

Economic evaluation

Progress on deciding what to spend on health care cannot be made without more precise data on productivity. This requires economic evaluation in which the costs of interventions are related to their benefits.

In the narrowest sense benefits can be measured in lives saved or life years saved, as in cost effectiveness analyses. In the widest sense these benefits can be measured in monetary units, as in cost-benefit analyses. Monetary estimates of benefits can be generated through willingness to pay techniques; but measures remain at present very experimental.[3] A more limited improvement to the use of narrow measures is the quality adjusted life years (QALYs) approach.[4] Limitations of QALYs should be recognised.[5 6] They are but part of the ever improving field of outcome measurement.

In any case, with decent data on outcomes, within the health care budget, resources could be allocated to those areas where health gains to the community are greatest relative to expenditure, ensuring maximisation of the community's health given the resources available.

Economic evaluation can also be used to aid decision making regarding the size of the health care sector. Given a fixed level of funding for services, presumably a cut off point could be established above which services are funded (at the margin) and below which they are not. Those arguing for increased funding would then be able to present such results to governments and say that by not giving a specified number of pounds extra for health services, a specified number of units of health will be sacrificed. Claims about harm to the community from a lack of funding or the need for more efficiency in health services would be more easily substantiated or dismissed.

As has been pointed out, we have a duty to measure the

effectiveness of health care in some form. If we do not have evidence that spending at a level of five times, three times, or twice a minimum level is beneficial is it surprising that cost cutting politicians choose the minimum level?[7]

Other sectors' contributions to health

Another point to bear in mind in endeavouring to determine where we go from here is that health care is but one factor through which health is improved or maintained. Would it be more productive in terms of health improvements to spend extra monies outside the health care system or within it? It may be that arguing for more health care resources is to the detriment of health if such resources are won at the expense of those resources being put into a more health productive area, such as education or housing.[8-11]

Once again the direction is one of searching for better measures of health outcome as well as evidence on the effects on health of not only health care but also investment in other health producing activities. It will then be possible to examine whether or not the greatest health improvements for the community will result from a larger or smaller budget for health care.

Conclusions

International comparisons of spending on health care are naive and unhelpful. There does not seem to be any point in refining a method of comparison that does not tell us what we want to know. The challenges for research and development are to continue devising measures of health gain and to increase the use of techniques of economic evaluation and analyses of determinants of health. This will not result in a uniform level of spending across countries but will help decide where increases and decreases in available resources are best targeted. If determining the size of the health care budget is not to be left in the hands of those providing unsubstantiated arguments in favour of expansion or cuts, the future for health care budget setting must, to a certain degree, rest with development of economic techniques.

1 British Medical Association. *Leading for health: a BMA agenda for health*. London: BMA, 1991.
2 Organisation for Economic Cooperation and Development. *Measuring health care—1960-1983, expenditure, costs and performance*. Paris: OECD, 1985.
3 Donaldson C. Willingness to pay for publicly-provided goods: a possible measure of benefit? *Journal of Health Economics* 1990;**9**:103-8.

4 Williams A. Economics of coronary artery bypass grafting. *BMJ* 1985;**291**: 326-9.
5 Donaldson C, Atkinson A, Bond J, Wright K. Should QALYs be programme-specific. *Journal of Health Economics* 1988;7:47-57.
6 Loomes G, McKenzie L. The use of QALYs in health care decison making. *Social Science and Medicine* 1989;**198**:1336-43.
7 Andersen TF, Mooney GH. *The challenges of medical practice variations*. Basingstoke: Macmillan Press, 1990.
8 Carstairs V, Morris R. Deprivation: explaining differences in mortality between Scotland and England and Wales. *BMJ* 1989;**299**:886-9.
9 Grossman M. The correlation between health and schooling. In: Terleck NE, ed. *Household production and consumption*. New York: National Bureau of Economic Research, 1975.
10 Corman H, Grossman M. Determinants of neonatal morbidity rates in the US: a reduced form model. *Journal of Health Economics* 1985;**4**:213-36.
11 Auster R. The production of health: an exploratory study. In Fuchs VR, ed. *Essays in the economics of health and medical care*. New York: Columbia University Press, 1985.

Manpower

STEPHEN BREARLEY

Manpower is accorded just two thirds of a page in the BMA's agenda for health,[1] yet its importance in the overall strategy of health care provision cannot be overemphasised. Many of the other issues discussed in the document have manpower consequences, not only for doctors but also for nurses, other professional groups, and ancillary staff. The NHS is the largest employer in Europe and some 70% of its budget is spent on salaries and wages. For these reasons alone manpower demands serious consideration by anyone intent on drawing up a blueprint for a health service in the year 2000.

The role of the NHS

In trying to predict the likely manpower requirements of the health services in the next century it is necessary to make an assumption about the role which they will be required to fulfil. The first page of *Leading for Health* recalls the fact that health services are but a part of a broader strategy for improving health, which also includes social services, community and occupational health services, public utilities, local authorities, and bodies concerned with health education.

The magnitude of public spending on health and its distribution between the various responsible bodies are likely to remain matters of controversy for the foreseeable future. The past decade has seen increasing interest in the prevention of illness as opposed to its treatment and in caring for patients in the community rather than in institutions. Unfortunately, both of these shifts are expensive in financial and manpower terms. The flagship of the government's preventive strategy—the United Kingdom breast cancer screening project—has been estimated to cost £4500 per life year saved and has substantially increased the demand on surgical and radiological services for localisation breast biopsy. Community care requires more carers than institutional care, and *Leading for Health* notes the decreasing proportion of informal carers—relatives, friends, and volunteers—relative to the numbers of elderly and mentally ill people. The NHS acts as a safety net for those who can no longer cope in the community and, as the population ages further, this aspect of its task is likely to increase.

There seems little scope for reducing the amount spent on the NHS or for reducing its role in the overall health strategy. The service has been in a state of almost perpetual financial crisis throughout the 1980s, with demand outstripping supply, persistent long waiting lists, and numerous stories reported by the media of apparently scandalous failures of provision. The BMA, most of the general public, and many managers believe that more should be spent on it. Improvements in community care, disease prevention, and health promotion do not lead to reduced demands on the health service, and they increase the demand for trained health professionals.

The NHS's other role of seminal importance is that of providing training for health professionals, including those who will subsequently work outside it. In the past such training has largely been acquired through service on an apprenticeship model and the numbers trained have been related to service needs. More educationally based programmes are slowly gaining ground in both medicine and nursing, and the role of the NHS as an educational resource must be recognised and supported if sufficient numbers of health professionals are to be available to meet all needs in the future.

Skill mix and changing roles

Concepts of what constitutes appropriate work for doctors, nurses, and other groups of health workers vary from country to country. In countries which have large numbers of doctors relative to the population, doctors may often be found doing work which, in Britain, would be carried out by others, such as those in hospital administration, pharmacy, rehabilitation and physiotherapy, and nurse education. Where doctors are scarce substantial amounts of treatment may be carried out by paramedical practitioners. The correlation between density of doctors and task allocation, however, is not exact. In the United States there are over 25 000 medical assistants, who, on the basis of two years' training, undertake such tasks as patient

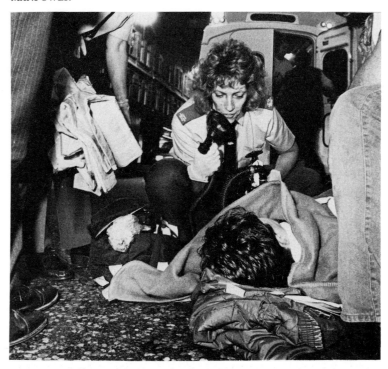

Paramedical staff work to a high standard and could take over some of doctors' duties

clerking, investigation, surgical assistance, and postoperative management, utilising written protocols. The accepted roles of doctors, nurses, and others in Britain are largely the result of tradition and bear re-examination.

Both the medical and the nursing professions have proved conservative in their attitudes to changing or extending roles, as evidenced by their opposition to the introduction of nurse prescribing, to the trial appointment of a paramedical surgeon's assistant in cardiothoracic surgery in Oxford, and to the giving of parenteral drugs by nurses. Yet in other areas non-medical staff have proved their value as counsellors, diagnosticians, and therapists. The need to reduce the burden on junior doctors has led to discussions between the BMA's Junior Doctors Committee (JDC) and the Royal College of Nursing on the reallocation of tasks, and the University of London has taken a lead in insisting on the presence of ward clerks and phlebotomists in hospitals whose house jobs it approves.[2]

Experience in the United States and elsewhere proves that appropriately trained paramedical staff can carry out many medical tasks to a high standard, and such staff are cheaper to train and employ than doctors. Not surprisingly, the possibility of introducing more paramedical staff is beginning to arouse interest in Britain. The scope for transferring substantial amounts of medical work to other groups is limited, however, by current demographic trends. The number of school leavers is currently in decline and the NHS is anticipating increasing recruitment problems over the next decade, particularly into nursing. An economic upturn is likely to exacerbate the problem, as prosperous private sector employers usually offer better salaries than the NHS. *Leading for Health* lists some of the reasons why the NHS may be considered an unattractive employer, including low pay, insufficient attention to training, poor incentives, long hours, a poor environment, high sickness and accident rates, and the absence of an occupational health service.

Although the implementation of Project 2000[3] may partially offset the shortage of nurses, there are grounds for serious concern about how wards, clinics, and operating theatres can be staffed at the turn of the century. Unimaginative and outdated personnel management policies will have to be substantially revised if recruitment and retention of staff of all grades and disciplines is to improve. At present there is no large, untapped pool of workers willing and able to take on substantial volumes of work formerly done by doctors.

Britain has one of the poorest ratios of doctors to population in the developed world,[4] and any attempt to replace doctors with other health professionals would make the disparity even greater, as well as being publicly and politically unpopular. Medical advances tend to lead to the introduction of treatments which are even more demanding on doctors' time than those they replace. Although some of the chores carried out by junior hospital doctors, especially house officers, could well be undertaken by people other than doctors, demand for medical skills remains high and is likely to grow. Unlike in the other health care professions there is no recruitment problem into medicine.

Medical manpower

The Department of Health's manpower tables show that hospital medical staff in Great Britain increased by 11% between 1985 and 1990 but, despite *Achieving a Balance*,[5] the ratio of juniors to seniors

79

barely changed and, in fact, deteriorated after 1987. The number of principals in general practice grew at almost exactly the same rate but began to decline again in 1989.

The 1989 report of the Advisory Committee on Medical Manpower Planning (ACMMP) suggested that the number of medical students emerging from British medical schools was sufficient to meet the country's needs for the time being. A crude calculation of the number of career posts becoming available annually (about 1200 in general practice, 700 in consultant practice, and a few hundred more in all other fields) suggested that there might, in fact, be difficulty in finding jobs for almost 4000 new graduates after their postgraduate training; but against this is the continuing low level of medical unemployment in Britain and the recruitment difficulties being experienced in some areas. Little information exists on the careers of the substantial number of doctors who do not follow conventional pathways, but some at least may be women who find current working practices incompatible with their other responsibilities and either stop practising altogether or work in intermediate level, non-training, and often part time posts.

The Advisory Committee on Medical Manpower Planning's figures have been superseded by a new study carried out by the Permanent Working Group of European Junior Hospital Doctors[6] as part of a survey of medical manpower in western Europe. This study looked at trends in supply and demand (defined as opportunities of medical work) over the past 20 years and made projections for the future. It concluded that Britain would remain self sufficient in doctors up to the year 2000 if demand were to grow at 1% per annum. Growth at just over 2% per annum, as has been seen recently, will leave the country over 6000 doctors short by the turn of the century.

These figures will certainly need to be scrutinised by the government's recently established standing committee on medical manpower.[7] If confirmed they suggest that a substantial and speedy increase in British medical school intakes is necessary, and even this will not avert a shortage because of the duration of basic and postgraduate medical training. In the medium term any shortage is likely to be made up by doctors from overseas, and especially from the European Community; but medical self sufficiency has been an aim of successive governments ever since the Todd report of 1968 and should remain so. It seems unjust to deny talented British school leavers the opportunity of pursuing a medical career when so many wish to do so and when there is clearly a need for their services.

80

It therefore seems likely that present trends in the demand for doctors, as indicated by the number of NHS posts established, will continue. But there is a need to increase medical staffing levels in the NHS even more rapidly. The responsibilities of NHS doctors have increased dramatically in the past few years. Resource management and the changes that have flowed from the white paper *Working for Patients*[8] have required hospital doctors to become more involved in management, while the widespread adoption of medical audit has been a further call on their time. Doctors are being urged, sometimes under threat of sanction, to devote more time to postgraduate and continuing medical education. Hospital stays are becoming shorter, turnover faster, and methods of treatment more demanding, all leading to more intensive working patterns. The recently published patient's charter imposes certain standards, particularly in respect of waiting times, which will increase the pressure on hospital doctors further.[9] Meanwhile, general practitioners have had to undertake new tasks and meet new targets as a result of their new contract. All these increases in activity have been introduced at a time when hospital medical manpower is growing at an underlying rate of barely 2% per annum and the number of general practitioner principals is actually declining.

That such demands cannot be sustained has perhaps been most clearly illustrated by the growing pressure for a reduction in junior doctors' hours of work. The reason that hours have become intolerable is not that they have become longer—they have not—but work has intensified to insupportable levels.[10] Sadly, the so called "new deal" for junior doctors,[11] agreed by senior doctors, juniors, the medical royal colleges, and the NHS management, fails to confront this issue. It will result in the same amount of work (or more) being done by a similar number of doctors in shorter hours at the cost of even more intensive working during periods of duty and what many see as unsatisfactory working arrangements (shifts and partial shifts). It is unlikely to boost junior doctors' flagging morale or to stem the growing tide of disillusioned senior house officers who are leaving medicine.[12]

The problems of excessive workload and long hours will be solved only by an increase in hospital medical staffing levels. This will require additional funding and therefore a political decision to be taken at high level. Because of the need to maintain a balance between numbers of senior and junior doctors expansion will have to be most rapid at consultant level, but more junior posts are also needed. In

81

future consultants will have to have a greater sessional commitment to emergency work and fewer fixed sessions.

Such changes are likely to be resisted by senior doctors, who have always reacted instinctively against an increase in their number, and by ministers, among whose primary concerns is constraining the NHS budget; but they are essential if acceptable standards of hospital care are to be maintained. Morale among doctors at all levels is low and substantial numbers are leaving the profession, diverting into non-clinical areas or retiring early. The workload of those who remain is unreasonable, particularly in view of the increased expectancy of leisure and family time in society generally. The achievement of satisfactory hospital medical staffing levels is, perhaps, the most pressing political challenge for the medical profession in the next 10 years. It is quite the most important issue to which the standing committee on medical manpower will have to address itself.

The sources of change

NHS employees are used to a service which is centrally planned and to negotiating with a single employer. Until recently staffing levels and personnel management policies have been determined nationally, with greater or lesser devolution of responsibility to operational units. This system is about to change with the growing numbers of NHS trusts. One of the freedoms given to trusts is the power to determine their own staffing structures and remuneration packages. The health departments, which have never been keen to impose staffing levels on health authorities, are likely to exert even less influence in future and the prospects of altering staffing levels through national agreement will recede.

It is still too early to assess the performance of trusts as employers. Some have already sought to make changes in the contracts issued to newly appointed consultants and they are likely to show interest in performance related pay, fixed term contracts, and a whole time commitment. This approach is likely to prove self defeating. In an era of staff shortage, which may be imminent, trusts may have to compete with each other in offering attractive packages. They will be wise to adopt some of the personnel management techniques of industry if they wish to recruit, retain, and motivate staff successfully.

Consultants are a good buy for trusts. Most are highly motivated, innovative, and work well beyond their contractual commitments. Their expertise makes them attractive to quality conscious purchasers of services. Senior registrars and registrars will remain employees of regional health authorities, with nationally negotiated terms and conditions of service and numbers regulated by the manpower committees. For all junior staff the training bodies have a considerable responsibility in ensuring that workload, hours of work, and staffing levels are reasonable and consistent with the educational purpose of their posts. They should not hesitate to withdraw recognition from posts where this is not the case.

Quality of service is becoming a real issue in the placing of contracts, and this should lead to more enlightened employment practices than have been evident in the past. Staff who feel valued and cared for are likely to be better motivated and to deliver a better service than those who are facing unreasonable demands in disagreeable surroundings.

1 BMA. *Leading for health: a BMA agenda for health.* London: BMA, 1991.
2 University of London. *Inappropriate duties for pre-registration house officers.* London: University of London, 1991.
3 United Kingdom Central Council. *Project 2000. The final proposals.* London: UKCC, 1987.
4 Schieber GJ, Poullier JP. Overview of international comparisons in health care expenditures. In: *OECD Social Policy Studies. Health care systems in transition.* London: OECD, 1990.
5 Department of Health and Social Security. *Hospital medical staffing: achieving a balance.* London: HMSO, 1987.
6 Permanent Working Group of European Junior Hospital Doctors. *Medical manpower in Europe. From surplus to deficit.* Bern: PWG, 1991.
7 Beecham L. Medical manpower review. *BMJ* 1991;**303**:1140.
8 Secretaries of State for Health, Wales, Northern Ireland, and Scotland. *Working for patients.* London: HMSO, 1989. (Cmnd 555.)
9 Department of Health. *The patient's charter.* London: HMSO, 1991.
10 Bulstrode C. Vice-versa: consultant becomes a junior. *BMJ* 1991;**303**:255-6.
11 NHS Management Executive. *Junior doctors. The new deal.* London: NHSME, 1991.
12 Allen I. *Doctors and their careers.* London: Policy Studies Institute, 1988.